SUPERNATURAL OUTCOMES; A SURGEON'S EYEWITNESS ACCOUNT

by Dana Edwards, MD,FACS

PROLOGUE

I am a board certified general surgeon with over 20 years experience; and I am a Christian. I meet people in the emergency department, not the sanctuary, my workbench is the operating table, not the pulpit, I smell human pus, blood, and excrement, not ceremonial incense, candle, or communion wine, my vestment is scrubs, not a ecclesiastical robe, I use a scalpel, not a baptistery, I suture wounds, dissect human organs, resect cancers, remove intestine, resuscitate the dead and dying, drain fluid, stanch bleeding, extricate gangrene, separate disease from human beings, and pray with and for patients. I am not a minister, pastor, lay leader, deacon, elder, church officer, or choir member; I am a surgeon first and a Christian second. That order of priority may offend some but I offer no apology. God ordained me to surgery just as surely as He ordained others to the ministry. Is anyone offended when a pastor says he is a pastor first and a Christian second? What God has ordained you to be is your ministry and the ministers outside the organized church and religious ministry provide the most powerful and impactful witness for God. The purpose of this book, besides telling a true and factual story, is to show how God uses all of us non-ministers in heroic ways. I certainly do not disparage ministry as a whole or ministers as a group, I only wish to make very clear that this book has no ministerial, religious, church, liturgical, or ecumenical agenda. After reading this book, I do not want you to attend my church, donate to my mission, volunteer for my cause, or give to my favorite charity. This is not a child book or a family book; it is a book full of horrors, humor, human suffering, tragedies, and death. It is not a spiritual teaching book; I offer no insightful scripture commentary. There are plenty of those books. My agenda is to show you what happened to theses patients exactly as I witnessed them so you become the surgeon. You examine the patients. You talk with the families. You review all the X-rays and labs and physical findings just as I did. Then, you take those patients into the operating room and see exactly what I saw; in other words, you become the eyewitness to events that simply should never happen in the twenty-first century; but they did.

I have changed all the names except mine and my surgical partner and life partner of over 20 years, my wife Angel. I have added nothing to the events except my thoughts as a surgeon. I have left nothing out except what my own memory may have inadvertently forgot. I have also changed some of the chronology to protect the privacy of the people I encountered.

A USUAL PRESENTATION

Patsy Conway loaded into the trunk of her 2001 Chevrolet Impala, thirteen, two foot high, one foot wide, blooming azalea bushes. She expertly and carefully arranged them side by side to form a blooming matrix that not only looked good but also closely bolstered each plant preventing them from tipping over during her 20 mile trip home to the goose rock community of Clay County Kentucky. It was an unusually hot Saturday morning for mid May in eastern Kentucky and she was determined to take advantage of it. " I'll get one extra just in case I damage one in transport or in planting," she thought as she paid the clerk for the bakers dozen.

Once she arrived home, she spent the rest of the sunny day digging up the old annuals from last spring and replacing them with the new azaleas. She had measured the length of her sidewalk from her garage to her back porch steps and knew the 12-foot length would allow her enough space to easily plant a half-dozen on each side of the slightly curving concrete sidewalk. After planting the last bush, she straightened her sore back and moaned just a little, "it just isn't any fun getting older," she whispered to herself. "Well, I did good. I didn't damage a single plant", she whispered again. But she still had the one azalea plant.

Next door, not 30 yards from Patsy's front door, stood the white clapboard farm house with the wide front porch and the large back yard and an even larger front yard. In the middle of the front yard, surrounded by a circle of tulips, decorated with a tire swing, and home to a dozen bird feeders, towered the century old black walnut tree; a tree Patsy had scraped her elbow climbing, broken two baby teeth swinging on its tire swing, and bruised her ribs when she fell out of it. She had spent her childhood under its canopy because she lived in that farmhouse with her mother and father as the only child of Georgia and Gabriel Conway.

While push mowing the front yard on a hot and humid late July day five years ago, Gabriel's heart stopped and Georgia's loneliness started. Despite Patsy living next door, Georgia's life became a routine of repetitive daily acts highlighted by a morning walk around the back yard garden and a late afternoon walk around the flowerbeds in the front yard. These routine undertakings, along with an assortment of house cleaning and laundering jobs, filled Georgia's days pretty well but it did nothing for her nights. At night, Patsy would help cook supper for the two of them and afterwards they would play a game of monopoly or rummy or work on patchwork quilts and cross stitching landscapes and farm scenes. Every Wednesday night, after church services at the Briar Creek Holiness church, they would ride over to London and eat at either Cracker Barrel or Shiloh's-the local steak restaurant. Patsy would take Georgia grocery shopping every other Friday at the Manchester IGA and then they would walk together in the memorial park. The activity really didn't matter to either, it was the routine of it that mattered; structured time was the defense against the relentless, incessant, and persistent gloom of despair and depression; and Patsy knew Georgia's routine and labored daily to keep it unbroken.

Patsy walked over to the walnut tree and began digging up some of the dark, rich, compost soil around the huge trunk. She planted the azalea bush and weeded some around the sunflowers and tulips and hydrangeas. A small patch of poison ivy clung to an exposed root and she quickly removed it using gloves and her trowel; Georgia and her both were extremely allergic to poison ivy and if they contacted the vine both would need a two week course of steroids. After finishing her gardening tasks, she stood up and looked at her watch: 6:45. She frowned and anxiously looked at Georgia's front door. "She is 15 minutes late for her walk," she thought to herself. She brushed off the dirt from her denim skirt, left her gardening tools and plant food by the tree and walked up to the front door.

When she walked into her childhood home she immediately heard the moaning. "Momma?" she yelled.

"In here. Living room." She replied in a weak staccato voice.

When she reached her, Georgia lay on her right side curled up with her knees bent toward her abdomen and her hands clutching the couch cushions. She was shaking, chilling, and moaning in pain.

"Momma! What's wrong? Where do you hurt? What's the matter?"

"I don't know. I hurt all over my belly. Worst pain I've ever had. Bad as birth pains. No, worse. At least labor would ease up for a while. This won't quit. Won't quit."

Patsy laid her hand on her mother's forehead. Her skin was hot, sweaty, flushed. "When did this start momma?" Patsy saw the pain and panic in Georgia's eyes.

"I ate lunch at 12:30. It started a few minutes after I ate. It started in the lower left side. Severe pain. Then I got sick. I threw up once. But pain got worse. I thought it was just something I ate. I have never had anything like this before. Never. Pain is everywhere. Constant. I tried to get to phone and call you. But moving makes the pain unbearable. If I lay still and don't move the pain will not get worse. If I try to move, it kills me. Then, just before you came over, I started chilling. I'm cold Patsy. I'm so cold."

Patsy went to the hall linen closet and retrieved a thick quilt Georgia's mother had made 50 years ago. She placed it over her. "I'm calling the ambulance momma. We have to get you to the hospital."

"Okay Patsy. Whatever will get rid of this pain. I can't take much more of it." She whispered and closed her eyes and took fast shallow breaths.

"Momma? Why are you breathing like that?"

"It hurts to take a deep breath."

"Where does it hurt?"'

"Everywhere."

By the time the ambulance arrived, Georgia would hardly talk and when she did it was a one or two word whisper.

"Momma?" Asked Patsy. She got no response. "The ambulance people are here. Do you understand?"

"Yes." She whispered.

Her initial vital signs showed a heart rate of 140, regular but with frequent irregular beats, blood pressure of 90/40, respiratory rate of 40, shallow breathing with an oxygen saturation of 80% on room air. Once the EMS started Georgia on oxygen, her saturation improved to 94%. Bobbie Chadwell, the paramedic, recorded in his notes, "elderly Caucasian female; pale, diaphoretic, chilling, temperature of 102 orally, rapid shallow breathing; in obvious distress."

"Please give her something for her pain." Begged Patsy. "Can't you give her something? Please."

"We can't." Answered Bobbie. " Her blood pressure's too low. She's dehydrated and septic. If I give her morphine, it could kill her. We're starting an IV and giving her fluids but no pain meds."

When the EMS unloaded her at the Emergency Department (ED), Georgia was able to talk in short sentences again and seemed more conscious. Her initial vital signs in the ED showed a heart rate of 120, regular, blood pressure of 100/60, oxygen saturation of 99% on 6liters of oxygen by nasal cannula, respiratory rate of 28 and a temperature of 101 orally.

Dr. Joseph Quinton, the ED physician working that evening directed the EMS to move her into the large trauma room 1-the room where he puts the sickest or most injured.

"What is your name please?" He first asked her.

Georgia raised her head and looked at the tall, thin, bald physician. She didn't like him. He didn't have a friendly face. "Georgia Ann Conway."

"Where do you hurt?" He raised his voice once he saw she was 79 years old.

"Everywhere in my belly. And I'm not deaf."

Dr. Quinton smiled slightly. "I'm sorry. I wasn't sure. When did the pain start?"

"This afternoon. Right after lunch."

"What time was that precisely?"

She disapprovingly looked at him again. "Lunch time. Noon. I started hurting at 12:30. You know. Right after lunch."

"On a scale of 1 to 10 where 10 is the worst pain you could imagine, where would you rate your pain?"

Georgia quickly answered, "15".

"I see. Are you hurting now?"

"Yes. It hasn't quit and it's getting worse."

"Why did you wait over 5 hours to get checked out?"

"I thought it would get better on its own. I"m not a doctor fan."

"Ever have pain like this before?"

"Never."

"Any other symptoms?"

"What do you mean?"

" Nausea, vomiting, chills, fever, diarrhea, shortness of breath, headaches, blurry vision, dizziness, hard time urinating?"

"Yes."

"What do you mean yes? Which symptoms have you had?"

"All of them."

Dr. Quinton audibly sighed.

"What medicines do you take daily?"

"Some. I'm not sure."

"Any blood thinners like aspirin or Coumadin?

"No."

"Heart disease or high blood pressure or thyroid disease or diabetes?"

"High blood pressure med."

"Drug abuse or alcohol abuse?"

Now she really disliked him, "No."

"Do you smoke or use tobacco at all."

"No."

"Any allergies?"

"Sulfur."

"Any surgeries in the past?"

"Two. Gallbladder and hysterectomy."

"How about appendectomy?"

"I don't think so."

"When did you have the gallbladder removed?"

"When Kennedy died. Old Dr. Reckner did it. He died years ago."

"When did you have the hysterectomy?

"61 years ago." Dr. Quinton stopped writing and looked at her.

"How do you know that so precisely?"

"It happened two days after my daughter was born. "Georgia disliked this doctor more and more.

"Any family with you?"

"My daughter, Patsy. She should be out in the waiting room. "Georgia's breathing became rapid and shallow again. The IV fluids were not running fast enough. And her pain was increasing.

"Doctor. I'm really hurting. Can I have something?"

He checked her latest vital signs. " No, your blood pressure is still too low." He slung his stethoscope from his neck and began his physical exam. In his ED note, he listed the following: head, ears, eyes, nose, and throat-within normal limits (WNL); lymphatic-WNL, lungs-clear. No wheezing. No crackles. Rapid breathing; heart- rapid with occasional dropped beat, no murmurs, no gallops, no rubs; abdomen-distended, tympanitic (bloated with a hollow air filled sound when he thumped it with his fingers), no bowel sounds, tender throughout to light palpation, rebound tenderness (severe pain when, after pressing down on the abdomen, he suddenly released the pressure), guarding (flinching when he pressed against the abdomen), and rigidity (involuntary tightening of the abdominal wall muscles)-all signs of peritonitis or severe infection inside the abdominal cavity. Well-healed right upper quadrant scar. Well-healed lower midline scar-both scars were narrow, smooth, and barely noticeable; rectal and genitalia-deferred.

Regina Robinson, RN was the ED nurse assigned to trauma room 1. She notes that after Dr. Quinton finished his exam and history, he instructed her to bolus a liter of normal saline, change her into a hospital gown, give a gram of a broad spectrum antibiotic through her IV, and allow her family into the room.

He ordered a series of tests including X-rays of her chest and a computerized axial tomography (CAT) of her abdomen and pelvis, complete blood count (CBC), comprehensive blood panel, urinalysis, arterial blood gas, EKG, and urine drug screen; he also called me to ensure I was available for a potential surgical case.

Regina finished the orders and brought Patsy into the room. Regina notes that Georgia's vital signs after the liter of fluid and the antibiotic had not changed significantly; she still had a systolic blood pressure in the 90's and a heart rate in the 100 to 120 range. Georgia urinated into a sterile collection jar and Regina noted how dark and concentrated the urine appeared.

"Momma?" Patsy called after standing next to the stretcher for a few seconds. Georgia opened her eyes and looked at Patsy.

"Momma. How do you feel?"

"Bad. I hurt Patsy and they won't give me anything for it."

"Regina. She says she's hurting. Can't you give her something?"

Regina explained to her the reasons why she could not give any pain meds.

"What's wrong with her?" Patsy held Georgia's left hand, rubbed Georgia's arm, and stared at the white, ashen, pale face. Georgia kept her eyes closed, her knees pulled up toward her chest, and her dry cracked lips parted slightly. Her tongue felt thick, immobile, almost paralyzed.

"We don't know yet." Regina had moved to Georgia's right side and checked the IV site. "We're waiting on the labs and X-rays to be completed. They should be coming any minute for the CT scan. I think Dr. Quinton did call the surgeon."

"Surgeon? Why?" Patsy looked at Regina for the first time.

"Just in case there is something a surgeon would need to fix. He's just making sure the surgeon is close by." Regina presented her best fake smile. But Patsy wasn't convinced.

"I don't want her to have surgery." Georgia moaned again and opened her eyes.

"Patsy. I'm hurting so bad. Please make them give me something. I'm thirsty too."

"Can she have something to drink?" Asked Patsy.

"No. Not yet. We have to complete the tests." Regina collected the urine to send to the lab and left the room. As she was leaving, the lab tech came in to draw the blood and behind her entered Levin Bradshaw, the X-ray tech. Patsy left and stood in the hall while Levin shot the three X-rays. While standing there, Dr. Quinton came up.

"Hello, I'm Dr. Quinton, the ED doctor today. Are you the family?"

"Yes. I'm Patsy Conway. I'm her only child."

"Does your mom live alone?" He asked in his monotone voice.

"Yes but I live right next door so I keep an eye on her. I didn't know anything was wrong until I found her at around 6:45."

"She ever have anything like this before?"

"No. Never."

"Where is your father?"

"He died. Five years ago. She never remarried. Can you tell me anything about what is wrong with her? The nurse said you had called a surgeon. Is that really necessary? What's wrong?"

"I'm not sure. I have some thoughts but nothing will be confirmed until the tests are all done. What I can tell you is there is something wrong in her abdomen and it appears to be some kind of infection and this infection has caused peritonitis, dehydration, and sepsis. The most common causes do require surgery to fix so I called Dr. Edwards." As he was talking to Patsy, he was slowly backing away down the hall. Patsy followed.

"I'm giving her IV fluid and antibiotics and as soon as her

blood pressure is normal, I can give her a little morphine" He kept slowly backing. Regina walked up with some sheets of paper.

"Hey Dr. Quinton. Here are the lab results and X-ray is here to take her for the CT scan." He audibly sighed and grunted, " Thanks Regina." He glanced down at the labs. Patsy walked beside the stretcher, holding her mom's hand. "I'm right here momma. I'll go with you for the X-ray."

After Dr. Quinton finished reading the labs, he asked Regina to call me and review them with me. "Tell him this is the usual presentation for a perforation." Said Dr. Quinton. When she called, I had just finished eating supper with my kids. After she finished reading them to me, I told her I was on my way. She told me the CT scan result wasn't back and then she told me Dr. Quinton's message. I told Angel we may need to do surgery but for her to stay home until I knew for certain. "I'll call you as soon as I know what we need to do."

When Georgia returned from the CT scan, her blood pressure was 110/83, heart rate of 109, and oxygen saturation of 94%. Regina injected 4 milligrams of morphine into her IV and Georgia went to sleep within five minutes. Patsy continued holding her hand, rubbing her arm, and watching her face. Finally, for the first time in many hours, her mother was pain free and resting. She watched her rapid, fast, and quiet breathing; she wasn't pleading for pain relief anymore. Patsy remembered, when she was 7 years old, she had one of her worst asthma attacks. Her parents rushed her to this same hospital, the only hospital in Clay county, and the doctor deposited her in a plastic, zippered oxygen tent and injected her with some type of medicine. It seemed to take hours before she could breathe without struggling. She was scared and it was the first time in her life that she thought about dying. Georgia had held her hand and sang her favorite song to her and Patsy remembered how that soft lullaby of a song had calmed her and reassured her. She bent over her mother, placed her face just a few inches from Georgia, and began softly singing.

"Hush little baby don't you cry. Papa's going to buy you a mockingbird. And if that mockingbird won't sing, Papa's going to buy you a diamond ring...."

Patsy rubbed the gold wedding ring on her momma's left ring finger. It was smooth and thinned out at places; Georgia told her at Gabriel's funeral, "death has separated our bodies, but not our souls. In my soul, I'll always be married to that man."

Patsy wanted to lower the head of the stretcher so Georgia would be in a more natural sleeping position but Regina wasn't in the room and she didn't know how to work the handles so she just continued holding Georgia's hand, rubbing her back and softly singing. She looked at her momma and realized for the first time how old she looked; how worn, fragile and weak she appeared. She rubbed her mom's forehead gently with her fingertips and felt the deep wrinkles. "I love you momma. I have always loved you. I love you so much." She felt the tears well up now and trickle down her face. But she couldn't stop. "Oh momma. I know you might die and I don't know what to do to help you. I don't know what to do. You have always helped me momma. What can I do?" She whispered out loud. She continued to talk to her in a low soft voice. "Momma, you remember the time you and daddy went out of town to celebrate your anniversary? You sent me over to aunt Ruby's and uncle Dick's to stay. I cried and cried. I must have been 10 but I cried anyway. I had never spent a single night away from you and daddy. Aunt Ruby tried to make me feel better. She and uncle Dick played card games, and red light, green light, and hide-and-go-seek. She made me homemade cookies and let me lick the icing bowl. She tried so hard to please me but all I wanted was you and daddy. I begged her to let me call you but she said no. She said you were on a honeymoon you never had. But I didn't care momma. I just wanted you so bad. I was just so selfish. When you called aunt Ruby to check on me, she almost didn't let me talk to you but I pitched such a fit that she finally gave me the phone. Oh momma. I'm sorry for that. I'm so sorry for ruining your trip with daddy. Please forgive me. You came home late that night and picked me up. You changed all your plans. You never went on that honeymoon trip. I wish, momma, I could go back and change that. You and daddy needed that trip and I messed it all up." If

Georgia heard what Patsy was saying, she didn't acknowledge it; she lay quietly sleeping. She still had a high heart rate, a mild fever, and rapid breathing but she wasn't hurting.

"If I don't get to tell you again momma, I want you to know how thankful I am to God for making you my momma. Nobody in the world ever had a better momma. You have always loved me even when I was bad. Don't die momma. Please don't die. Please."

Then Patsy prayed out loud; her first prayer that day, " dear God in heaven. Sweet Holy Jesus. Cure her. Please cure her. Send someone to cure her; send your Holy Spirit, I'm just not ready to be alone. Please Father, don't let her die."

I stood a few feet behind her and listened to her plead to God; it was unlike the pastors' and ministers' prayers. Her words flowed out, uninterrupted, in a stream of syllables, undisturbed by the clergy's cacophonous repetition of 'Father' or 'Lord' or "ah". Her words depicted the image of her heart, a heart in turmoil and turbulence; displayed a life turned topsy-turvy; and disclosed a soul in terrible trouble and torment. Only a human being in great anguish and despair could pray like her. If the prayer in Gethsemane had been recorded, it must have sounded something like Patsy's prayer that May night.

I cleared my voice. "Excuse me." She didn't turn around but she stopped praying. "I'm Dr. Edwards, I'm the surgeon here in town." She turned slightly to the right and looked at me with her right bloodshot eye, covered by a swollen eyelid and blurred by a pool of tears.

"I'm Patsy Conway. This is my mother, Georgia Conway." She said this with pride like a parent introducing herself to a group of spectators at her child's piano recital.

"I'm so sorry to meet you like this. I see your mother is very ill so I'll just ask you a few questions. I talked with Dr. Quinton and looked over his notes and labs and things. Uh, I've just looked at the CT scan results as well." I waited for her response but she had turned back to look at her sleeping mother; she didn't speak at all.

"Do you know what her first symptom was and when it

occurred?

"I don't know. I found her at around 6:45 lying on her couch in terrible pain. She was hurting in her belly but she didn't tell me anything else." Her voice was low, deep, hoarse like she had just finished a singing performance for a Wagner opera.

"Has Dr. Quinton told you anything about her condition or diagnosis?"

"Said it was some type of infection and that he may call a surgeon, you I guess, and that he's waiting on some tests results."

"Okay. All that is true. Now I need to examine your mother so I'll have to wake her. You can stay while I examine her." I told her this as I gently shook Georgia's curled legs and spoke her name. She opened her eyes and looked first at Patsy and then her eyes met mine. Her eyes, surrounded by deep furrows and wrinkles, looked clear, but weary. The pupils were small with a narrow ring of white pigment around them; arcus seniles. She squinted slightly and asked in a whisper, " Who are you?"

"I'm Dr. Edwards Mrs. Conway. I'm the surgeon that Dr. Quinton called to check you out."

"Oh. That grumpy ED doctor. Why'd he call you?"

"He thinks you may have something wrong that will require me to fix. But I'll have to examine you to make sure. Do you mind Mrs. Conway?"

"No. But call me Georgia. My mother-in-law was Mrs. Conway. I'm Georgia." I thought I saw a slight smile.

"Okay Georgia. I'll just close this curtain so we can have some privacy. Patsy can stay." I pulled the curtain around the bed but it was too short and could only shield one side of the bed. I lifted the blue, yellow polka-dot hospital gown and looked at her abdomen. It was pale white, smooth, and bloated like the underbelly of a frog. But it was not unmarked. Two separate but similar scars marred its otherwise silky surface. One ran under the natural protuberance of the lower right rib cage and extended from the midline to well past the edge of the ribs-a typical gallbladder surgery scar from at least 40 years ago. The other, and even less noticeable scar, coursed straight down the middle of the lower abdomen starting at the belly button and ending at the pelvic bone-the typical hysterectomy or caesarean surgery scar from, again, at least 40 years ago. Both scars were ancient and illuminating; their smoothness, faintness, and paleness, like a fossil, aged them like carbon dating and their length and size, like the excavated remains of an Egyptian tomb, represented a bygone surgical era when the size and length of incisions demonstrated the surgeons' need for exposure of vital organs and ease of dissection rather than the comfort and aesthetic desires of the patient.

I firmly laid my left middle finger against the mid abdomen and struck the middle finger with my right second and third fingertips evoking a hollow, drum like sound reminiscent of striking antediluvian half-filled water jars for primitive music. But in Georgia's case, if there was music present in the sound, it was the sound of an ominous jungle drum announcing the inevitable and early arrival of warriors of death.

But my thumping didn't just evince an air-filled sound; it also raised a scream of pain. My quick staccato finger thrusts against her abdomen shook her abdominal cavity, a cavity lined with a thin transparent film of nerve endings called the peritoneum. When those nerve endings become inflamed by any chemical or bacteria, moving them, even a millimeter, will evoke pain as severe as a blowtorch cauterizing the open exposed end of an amputated limb.

I gently and slowly laid my stethoscope on her lower abdomen and listened. The abdominal cavity is an orchestra of sounds; only in death, like a grave, is it totally silent. But the different sounds, their pitch, tone, and volume, their variations in musicality, their rhythm, pace, and syncopation, their crescendo and decrescendo, their bruits, and murmurings, in solos, trios, quartets, and quintets, reveal the presence or absence of many different diseases, pinpoint the location of narrowed, plaque filled arteries, determine the size of the liver, spleen, uterus, and bladder, and identify the displacement of the intestines into hernia pockets.

I listened for a full minute. I could hear the abnormal, distinct rhythmic swish of blood in both flanks but not in the midline or pelvic areas revealing diseased, narrowed kidney arteries but not the main abdominal arteries. I could hear her breath sounds because the gas exchange in the lungs fully transmitted through the thin diaphragms showing she had no fluid around or in the lungs. I could hear the heart sounds because the blood flow across the heart valves, through the heart chambers, and out the great vessels traveled unimpeded by weak, incompetent, leaking valve leaflets, moved unhampered by dilated, flabby, nonfunctional, ventricles or atriums, and passed straight through uninhibited by aberrant side currents and eddies through deviant holes and passages.

But it was what I didn't hear that alarmed me. I couldn't hear the gurgling, sloshing, bubbling yellow-green, enzyme laden, protein rich, fat infused, carbohydrate burdened intestinal fluid splashing along the hollow bowels, peristaltically pulsed, pushed and prodded toward the gaseous cavernous colon; the absence of bowel sounds provides clear evidence of bowel paralysis. This absence of serpentine movement predictably and inevitably follows the presence of infection, inflammation, and irritation; it is the first normal function to cease when the abdominal cavity is invaded by any alien substance or entity such as pus, bacteria, stool, intestinal fluid, blood, urine, or gastric acid. Silence in the abdomen is not golden.

I replaced the stethoscope into my lab coat pocket, pulled the gown back over her abdomen, and looked at Georgia and then at Patsy. They both stared back and waited. I cleared my voice, "Georgia, I have to tell you some very bad news. Do you understand?"

She quickly looked at Patsy and then back at me, "Yes. I understand." Her voice, audible but weak, did not demonstrate any impaired judgment.

"I don't know any other way to tell you other than just the blunt truth. Listen to me carefully and when I'm finished please ask me to clarify anything you don't fully understand." I sighed and cleared my voice again. Patsy stood holding Georgia's hand and faced me across the stretcher. Georgia looked hard at me.

"Your white cell count is 19,000 which usually indicates some type of serious infection. Your temperature is well over a 100, again consistent with infection. Your hemoglobin and hematocrit are both elevated, your sodium is high, and your urine specific gravity is 1.030, all indicating dehydration. Your CT scan showed free air, thickened sigmoid colon, some fluid accumulation in both sides of your pelvis. This means you have some perforation or hole somewhere inside you and that hole is leaking out infection which is poisoning your peritoneum and causing peritonitis. The scan cannot localize where the hole is, it just confirms the presence of peritonitis due to some rupture inside you. When I examined you, you have what we call peritoneal irritation signs such as no audible bowel sounds, severe tenderness called rebound tenderness and rigidity which is an involuntary abdominal wall muscle contraction in order to protect your abdomen from anything that might make the infection worse." I looked again at them but they both stayed silent.

"Now that we know what's wrong and that most likely the perforation occurred right after you ate lunch, which was roughly seven hours ago, we really must operate ASAP. In other words, we don't have much more time to save your life. You have to have an operation. I must explore your abdominal cavity, find the hole, close it, remove or repair the disease that caused the hole, wash out the infection, and get you off the operating room table as fast as possible. In addition, I need to place a large IV line into the main chest vein that lives underneath your collarbone. This line will enable me to draw blood, give medications, and infuse fluids and blood as needed."

"You think she will need blood?" Asked Patsy.

"I don't know for sure but I hope for the best and prepare for the worst. I really won't know what I need to do until I operate. This operation could take an hour or many hours. I may just need to suture a gastric ulcer hole closed and wash out the acid or I may even need to remove intestine or make a colostomy. So, I need your permission, Georgia to operate. Now, since you had some narcotics, Patsy will legally need to sign the permit but you need to give me verbal consent. Do you have any questions?"

I paused but neither spoke. "I must also, by law and by professional mandate, discuss the potential complications. This is not an exclusive list but only represents some of the more important and most dreaded complications. I'm not trying to scare you but reality is reality. This is a big major operation on a 79 year old so of course it carries risks." I paused again but no response.

I continued. "The complications of placing the central IV line include collapse of the lung, rupture of a major blood vessel, infection, and even death. The complications of a major abdominal exploration include heart attack, stroke, abscess, pneumonia, blood clots, wound infection, need for repeat surgeries, and of course death."

Georgia and Patsy looked at each other. Neither talked. "I'll leave you for a few moments. I'll go get Regina she we can get the permit signed. I'll be back shortly."

"I like him Patsy. He has a nice face. An honest face. I think I'll let him go ahead."

"Well whatever you say mom but we really don't know him. Of course, we don't have much of a choice. I'll sign it." As she said this, she leaned on the stretcher side rails slightly moving the bed. Georgia screamed in pain.

"I'm sorry momma. I'm so sorry. I didn't mean to. I'm sorry."

Georgia began breathing rapid again, her heart rate increased to 130 and her blood pressure dropped below 100; the morphine had worn off. Regina rushed in but by that time Georgia had quit screaming.

"What happened?"

"Momma is hurting again. Can you give her some more morphine?"

Regina checked her vitals again; blood pressure was 90/40, heart rate back up to 150. "We can't Patsy. Her blood pressure is too low again. Did you finish talking to Dr. Edwards? Are you ready to sign the permit?"

She didn't hesitate, "Yes and yes. Is Dr. Edwards coming back in before he starts the surgery?"

Regina witnessed Patsy's signature on the permit and then answered her," I 'll go tell him you need to see him." After she had left, Patsy watched her mother intently. She was breathing rapid and shallow again, wrinkling her forehead in pain, and the heart monitor was beeping fast and loud. I came into the room a few minutes after Regina talked with me. Pasty did not hear me again.

"Patsy? Do you have any questions? The OR team is ready. We need to go now." I was hoping she caught the urgent desperation in my voice; she didn't. She kept holding Georgia's left hand.

"Dr. Edwards?" she whispered hoarsely.

"Yes Patsy."

"Momma is hurting again. Could she have some more morphine?"

I sighed and gently shook my head. I stared at the back of this tall, thick bodied, broad shouldered only child of a dying mother. Patsy's long gray streaked black hair was piled up in a mass of bobby pins and hair spray and the skin on the back of her exposed neck was tan, smooth, and without any visible moles, or skin lesions; it was perfect for a deep blue, low collared, sleeveless, evening dress; a dress I knew patsy did not own, never had owned, and never would own. She was a woman content with who she was and not concerned with who she wasn't. She was the cashier at the local Wal-Mart, a member of the church singing group, an excellent piano player who plays by ear but can't read a single bar of written music, a gardener of vegetables and flowers, a quilt maker, an experienced and aggressive rook player, a reader of Jane Austen and the Bronte's, a Sunday school teacher, a spinster, and the only child of Georgia Conway; this last fact defined her the most, and I had guessed as much by hearing her prayer. I knew she was desperate to do something, anything, to help her mother. She couldn't direct her care, place the IV's, draw up the medications, run the fluids, order the tests, or perform the operation; but she could try to ease her mother's pain. It was the only loving, caring, kind act she could perform and she persisted in it.

"Patsy." I laid my hand on her shoulder. "We are going to take her to the operating room and the anesthetist will put her immediately to sleep and your mother will be out of pain."

Patsy looked at me, really looked at me for the first time. Her hazel eyes searched my eyes like a miner looking for gold in an unknown craggy, rock strewn, boulder covered, dry plain. "Dr. Edwards, will she die?"

How do you answer such an honest, desperate question, a question both seeking and revealing. She wanted the truth but her heart was breaking because she already knew the answer.

"Yes Patsy. She might very well die no matter what we do. I just don't know for sure but I'm sure about this, if we don't operate, she will die." Then she asked me something I was prepared for but not expecting.

"Will you pray for her?" Her eyes met mine again but this time they were not seeking for gold, they were pleading for hope.

I didn't answer. I grabbed her hand in my left hand, laid my right hand on Georgia's forehead, bowed my head, closed my eyes, and prayed the prayer I want prayed for me; the same prayer I have uttered for all these twenty years of operating. It comes from the gospel of John, chapter 9. "Dear Heavenly Father. Thank you for your son Jesus, for your love, for your mercy, for your grace, and for your power. I now lift up my sister Georgia. You made her. You created her. You love her. Now at the time of her greatest need, I pray every medication, every instrument, every hand, every device, every person, who touches her body be anointed with your healing holy spirit. Guide my mind, bless my hands and the hands of my assistants, and use whatever is needed, whatever you deem necessary to heal her, to prevent all complications, to restore her to perfect health. In the mighty name of Jesus. Amen"

CHAPTER 2

THE OPERATING ROOM

On that May night, the nurse anesthetist, Sonya Grubb, was on call. Over the last several years, Sonya and I had worked together on numerous cases at two different hospitals and she had provided the anesthesia on some of my most complicated and challenging cases; and yet I had never seen her upset, overwhelmed, or even slightly stressed; not even on the night of the shotgun blast.

A couple of years ago, about 9 in the evening, the ED physician called me frantically asking for help to stabilize a shotgun injured patient for air transport to the University of Kentucky trauma service. He didn't tell me on the phone that the victim was an 18-year-old boy nor did he tell me that another 18-year-old boy had shot him. When I arrived and rushed into trauma room 2, I couldn't see the patient because his stretcher was completely hidden by a mob of scurrying medical personnel. Joe Winters, a 400 pound EMT, was standing on the victims' left side, leaning on him, his flabby, hairy arms fully extended, and sweat dripping off his forehead and nose, performing some type of chest compressions. The ED physician, Dr. Geoffrey Bartel, stood on his right side, repeatedly jabbing a 3 inch long needle underneath his right collar bone in a desperate and frenetic attempt to find the completely collapsed and empty subclavian vein. Two respiratory therapists stood above his head; one squeezing 100 percent oxygen down an endotracheal breathing tube, while the other, to prevent the tube's dislodgment, tightly gripped, with both hands, the tube just above his lips. Two nurses were gathered around his outstretched arms attempting to aspirate blood for the lab and start two peripheral IVs. Two lab techs rested against the back wall waiting for the blood samples and holding six units of O negative untyped blood Dr. Bartel had ordered for emergency transfusion. Two radiology techs, slouched against their shopping cart sized portable X-ray machine, waited for Dr. Bartel's direction. And the pale, thin, victim, draped under a wispy white cotton shroud, lay motionless, silent, corpse like, sprouting a mangled, purplish-black mass of flesh in the center of what, less than an hour ago, had been his flat, washboard abdomen.

Of all the hospital emergencies, it is the gunshots, knifings, bomb blasts, impalements, dog bites, animal attacks, and any other violent act that breaks the skin, that requires the expertise of a general surgeon. A bleeding wound anywhere on the body will reflexively demand a call to the general surgeon. The injury could be as minor as a profusely bleeding scalp abrasion or as serious as a gunshot to the heart; doesn't matter, the general surgeon will be called.

After I arrived, Dr. Bartel quickly turned around and walked out. His medical experience and training did not prepare him for anything close to the severity of this boy's injury. But before he left he quickly told me a few pertinent facts.

"The family is out in the waiting room. Weirdest damn thing I've ever seen. One side of the room is this boy's family and the other is the shooter and his family. Now, get this Edwards. If this ain't the damnedest mess I've ever seen. The boy here and the shooter are first cousins. Right? Right. Tonight, after eating supper, they sat in this kid's front porch swing talking basketball, talking about who was the greatest player to ever play for Kentucky. One of the boys thinks its Richie Farmer and the other says Kyle Macy. Well, after a little while the discussion turns into a full-blown argument. I mean a real hollering match, at least according to this kid's family. Now, the other kids family says that what happens next is purely accidental. They say their kid goes to his truck and gets his new shotgun to show the other kid. You know, just showing what a great gun he has; just showing off. But, he didn't realize it was loaded with buckshot and when he laid it in the porch swing, the damn thing gets caught on the swing chain and goes off accidentally. Now, this kid's family says something totally different. They say they could hear'm both start yelling at each other for a few minutes and then they see the shooter run to his truck, whip out a 12 gauge shotgun, hurry back up on the porch, stop three feet away from this kid, holding the damn thing waist high like a fricking handgun, and fires the thing into this kids abdomen. I mean shit. A damn stupid argument about some old guys who played basketball decades ago; basketball? Go figure. Well, anyway, good luck."

At the same time I arrived, Sonya and the OR techs also arrive. Sonya secured the endotracheal tube, I placed a three lumen central line into the left subclavian vein, and started transfusing the blood. Sonya placed two more IVs into his arms, and the OR techs covered the abdominal wound with normal saline moist sterile gauzes and towels. Once we start the blood transfusions, infuse the IV fluids, and inject the epinephrine, his pulse and blood pressure return enough to know he is still alive but he is certainly not stable to transfer down the hall much less to a hospital 100 miles away, so we rush him into the operating room hoping we can at least stop the bleeding and get him stable enough to transfer.

Once in the OR, the entire team, Angel, Oma Phillips LPN, Constance Barkly ORT, Sonya, Cheryl Sevens RN, the circulating nurse, and myself, lifted him onto the OR table.

I told Jayme Eversole RN, the extra circulating nurse willing to come in and help, to pour the disinfectant, betadine, on him from his neck to his knees. "Do you want a Foley?" She asked.

"No. We don't have time. Sonya, what's his vitals?"

"No detectable blood pressure but I can feel a carotid pulse."

We squirted alcohol over our hands and forearms, gowned, gloved, and draped the patient in less than a minute; then we really looked at his wound. He had a large blast injury causing a grapefruit sized hole just to the right of the belly button. Several small buckshot puncture wounds tattooed the hole edges as well. Multiple segments of ripped and tattered large and small intestines cascaded, entwined, and coiled out along each side and continued down on top of his lower abdominal wall. Mixed in this intestinal ooze were light brown stool, green bile stained fluid, pieces of white corn and dark meat, and on top of it all quivered the gelatinous, red and purple blob of clotted blood. The disgusting odor of clotted blood, the offensive stench of feces, the stink of intestinal fluid, and the effluvium of methane and other bacterial gases, turned the OR air into a putrid, nauseating, repugnance.

I cut the skin above and below this fleshy crater, opened it up five inches above and below, scooped the intestinal residue into a tight ball and pushed it over to the left side of the abdominal wall; this obvious injury, as horrific as it was, was not killing this boy. It was something else; something deeper, vastly more serious, and immensely less odorous. To gain visualization of the injury, I shoveled the clotted blood out of the abdominal cavity. The multiple buckshot pellets, diffused throughout this clot, scraped against my gloved hands as I mucked it out and threw it into a large plastic basin. Some of the shot tore holes in my thin latex gloves forcing me to change gloves several times. All of this clot was old, no new blood flooded the area; there wasn't enough circulating blood left to extravasate.

At the bottom of the abdominal cavity, underneath the clot, against the backbone, just below the liver, to the left of the right kidney, to the right of the aorta, near the head of the pancreas, away from the spleen, remote from the diaphragm, distant to the stomach, I found the killing wound, the injury no surgeon could repair. The pellets and packing and gunpowder ripped out a 6 inch long segment of his inferior vena cava(the largest vein in the body, the vein responsible for collecting and returning all the blood below the diaphragm back to the right heart), tore out a 2 inch segment of the right kidney artery, pulverized the right kidney, obliterated the right adrenal gland, destroyed the right ureter, and shredded the paraspinal muscles. Within a few minutes after this injury, his entire blood volume, all 12 pints, spewed into his abdominal cavity, poured out the blast hole, washed across his macerated intestinal remnants , streamed over his genitalia, thighs, and buttocks, and finally pooled onto the brown porch boards; technically he was dead before the ambulance ever loaded him but legally he died ten minutes after I found the unrepairable wound.

We moved Georgia over to the narrow, thin cushioned, stainless steel OR table. The table is six feet long, cantilevered on a broad base allowing five feet of free space underneath for fluoroscopy. Once on the table, Shana Crawford RN, the circulating nurse, secured a thin, wide, black belt across her legs just below Georgia's knees and strapped her arms onto cushioned metal arm boards with thin, flexible, Velcro bands. "Arms to her sides?"

"No Shana. Arms out." I answered.

For most surgeries, particularly exploratory surgeries, the patient is posited in a recumbent supine position, legs straight and uncrossed, arms at 90 degrees, head straight, and back flat. If viewed from the ceiling, the position resembles either a crucified victim just before the executioners raise and drop them into the hole or a victim after the crucifixion is completed but just before removing the body. It is the position symbolizing sacrificial submission, total trust, and consummate confidence and it disturbs me. Once anesthetized, she is naked, exposed, defenseless, insentient and extremely vulnerable. Shana works fast to complete her checklist of safety protocols like ensuring the presence and proper placing of padding, visualizing grounding pad placement, safe and proper position of arms, identification of patient by birthdate, social security, hospital number, and name, verifying the written agreement between the signed permit and the proposed procedure, listing all allergies, recording the time the patient entered the room, time anesthesia started, and later, the time the surgeon makes the first incision, inspecting all IV sites for functionality, inspecting and recording room temperature and humidity to insure both follow strict guidelines, placing the intermittent compression boots on her legs to minimize the risk blood clot formation, confirming the proper use of preoperative antibiotics, clipping, by using an electric razor, all hair from the operative field , surveying the patient for acceptable surgery attire, and disinfecting and sterilizing the skin, and she does this all before I can make one incision; it is an exhaustive task but she is mandated to complete it during every operation, elective or emergent, during day shift hours or during late night or early morning hours, regardless of the situation, circumstance, or surrounding events.

As Shana, 6 months into her first pregnancy, finished her checklist, the OR techs also completed theirs. After positioning a 3-foot wide, 8-foot long stainless steel 'back' table a few feet from Georgia, they cover it with a double layer of sterile sheets large enough and long enough to hang over the edge 2 feet. Once sterilely covered, the techs open the rectangular surgical steel, steam sterilized deep instrument trays, remove all the implements needed, including instruments, needles, sutures, and sterile towels and sheets, and place them in prescribed rows. The particular instruments vary, but arrangement on the 'back' table is constant. Thus my 'back' table in Manchester hospital is identical to the 'back' table in Chicago, New York, and San Francisco; it is universal. This uniformity ensures every member of the surgical team will know the exact location of every instrument. But its purpose is not convenience, but rather productivity; fumbling to find a curved hemostat or long Vanderbilt or Kelly clamp or Lahey or DeBakey forceps will decrease efficiency, increase operative time, and therefore, decrease the number of surgeries a surgeon can complete before 3pm. If a surgeon goes past 3pm with elective cases, the hospital has to pay overtime to the OR staff and this will decrease profit margin since insurance reimbursement is solely based on the diagnosis and the exact operative procedure, not on operative time. A hernia repair that takes three hours will garnish the same pay as a 30 minute hernia repair; speed in the operating room is the ultimate goal and anything and everything that may slow the surgeon and extend the operative time, will be eliminated.

In the center of the back table, just in front of the instruments, the techs arrange packs of 18 by 18 inch square white cotton lap sponges; each pack contains five separate lap sponges and sewn onto the corner of each dangle six inch long thin blue radiographic ribbons like windless kite tails. Stacked near these lap sponges are similar, but much smaller, four by four inch square cotton sponges, called 4 by 4's, and braided through the cotton matrix of each of these stretches a double row of thin radiographic strings; each stack of 4 by 4's contain a dozen or more. These radiographic marked sponges might and do get "lost" in the abdominal cavity during an exploratory surgery, but an X-ray in the operating room will always find them.

After unpacking each tray of sterilized items and arranging them as prescribed on the back table, the techs audibly count each item and the circulating nurse writes the number next to the item on a printed checklist; this is called the preoperative instrument and sponge count and the techs complete this before the patient is brought into the operating room. The preoperative count is performed without any distractions. The nurse and techs keep the operating room door shut, discourage unnecessary entrance into the OR room, shut off all digital devices, and prohibit music; the entire count is in as near total silence as possible and only the techs and the circulating nurse are allowed to finish this task; it must be accurate and precise. No surgeon will close the incision until the needle, instrument, and sponge count is verified correct twice.

The techs that May night were BJ Sizemore and Jason Naples; both experienced but very different. BJ, a tall, thin African American, was talkative and gossipy. He enjoyed discussing other surgeons and employees and he took great pleasure in being the first to disclose some embarrassing or humorous story about anybody including surgeons; no topic or subject was off his list. Divorces, affairs, pregnancies, miscarriages, bankruptcies, diagnoses, drug and alcohol use, wild parties, car accidents, and job firings and hiring's were all exciting subjects for BJ. He served as the main source for personnel news in the surgery department. Everyone knew that a secret once told to BJ would cease to be a secret within 30 minutes. He was also the lunch clock aficionado.

After clocking in for work, he would immediately take the elevator to the second floor cafeteria, order breakfast, read and memorize the lunch menu, return to the surgery department and announce the items he would order for lunch. Although the cafeteria opened for lunch at 10:45, BJ would always wait until 10:50 before retreating back to the cafeteria for lunch; he said he never wanted to be the first in line, just the second.

Jason, an obese, eager to please, never argumentative, and quiet twenty-four year old, loved working in surgery and frequently volunteered for extra call. He was married, but not happily, and the father of two young children. He stayed in constant marital trouble because he regularly chose fishing and hunting over going home. He stored his guns and his fishing rods in his car because, " you just never know Doc when you might need them," he told me numberless times.

Both techs, despite their personality differences, knew their jobs and performed them well. Both had assisted me in hundreds of typical, common surgeries like appendectomies, cholecystectomies, colectomies, hernia repairs, skin cancers, skin grafts, amputations, abscess draining and endoscopy; they were not novices. After so many cases, we trusted each other. I trusted them to stay alert, focused, and engaged and they trusted me to operate fast, efficient, and competently.

Once Sonya had Georgia intubated and completely anesthetized, I twisted two non-sterile white bath towels into a tight roll, placed it vertically down the center of her back to elevate her shoulders and open the anatomical space between her collar bone and fist rib where the large chest vein, the subclavian vein, lies. This maneuver increases the chance of successfully placing the central line. I prep her chest skin, blindly push a large 4 inch long needle into the opened space and hope the vein is in the usual position. If the vein is out of position or the space does not open up or the lung is higher than normal or scar tissue is present or the collar bone has been fractured or the first rib doesn't exit or the presence of a dozen other abnormalities, then my attempt to place the IV line will not only fail but will collapse her lung, puncture her vein or artery, sever the catheter tip releasing it into the heart, cause a blood clot or air bubble to travel to her brain; any one of these complications will kill her. Placing central lines are common procedures for interns and are simple, uncomplicated, and extremely dangerous. By the time I finished my five years of surgery training in Johnson City, Tennessee, I had successfully completed hundreds of central lines but after 20 years of surgery practice and thousands of central line placements, I still cringe, sweat, and hyperventilate in a Pavlovian response to every request for a central line. And no matter how many I have placed, I would rather remove a perforated appendix, a gangrenous gallbladder, a hemorrhaging spleen, an infected leg, or a fungating, ulcerated skin cancer than place a central line. I can directly, visually, and actively treat, control, and repair any complication from the above listed surgeries and dozens more, but I cannot quickly, immediately, or successfully repair, resolve, or reverse most central line complications; they simply scare the piss out of me.

After finishing the central line, Shana frog legged Georgia's legs to expose her vulva, opened a sterile kit filled with the items needed to place the silicon, balloon tipped, flexible tubing down the urethra and into the bladder, wiped the vulva and urethral opening with three different betadine swabs, lubricated the tubing with thin clear jelly, pushed it forward until urine spilled into the tubing, pushed a syringe full of normal saline into the balloon preventing inadvertent removal, connected it to a 1000ml plastic collecting reservoir, taped the tubing to the underside of her right thigh, and transferred it to Sonya for her to measure, monitor, and manage during the procedure.

"How does the urine look?" I asked her as I headed toward the sink.

"Clear. Non-bloody. Not concentrated and so far about

500ccs but more is coming."

I stopped and looked back at Sonya. I walked back to her area at the head of the patient and looked in the urine bag; it was clear, dilute, non-bloody, and copious. "Get a set of vitals for me before you put down the NG tube."

She stopped opening the bag containing the nasogastric tube (NGT) and complied. "Blood pressure 134/84, heart rate 85, oxygen saturation 100% on 30%, and temperature 97.0." She answered quickly and then looked at me. I stared at her. "Are you sure?"

"I'll recheck." She did with the same results.

"How much fluid have you given?"

"I've given a liter since coming in and she got two liters in the ED."

"Well I guess you have done a great job of resuscitating. Go ahead with the NG and I'll check placement when I get in." I walked out with Angel to scrub.

Peritonitis paralyzes the stomach and intestines preventing contraction of the intestinal muscles, causing the intestinal fluid to stagnate instead of steadily moving toward the anus. This stagnation promotes bacteria overgrowth, boosts gas formation, distends the stomach and intestine, escalates vomiting of fecal smelling fluid; when the nurses smell this type of vomitus, they describe it as vomiting up stool. To prevent this inevitable event, Sonya stretches out a 4 foot long clear plastic tube called a nasogastric tube or NGT. She rubs lubricating jelly on the last 12 inches, curves the tip into a 30 degree angle, advances it into the right nostril, shoves it toward the back of Georgia's head until she meets resistance and then she nudges it forward a centimeter at a time until the resistance ends. At this point, the tip is leaning against the back of the throat dangling just past the tonsils, waiting to be pushed either too far forward so it enters the trachea and main windpipe or backwards and into the esophagus. Entrance into the first hole will cause coughing and possible dislodgment of the breathing tube and entrance into the second hole will allow passage into the stomach and accomplish the critical evacuation of stagnant gastric fluid full of acid and enzymes and possible food particles. Failure to pump all this fluid and food out of the stomach can lead to vomit entering the windpipe resulting in pneumonia, pneumonitis (inflammation of lung tissue), respiratory failure, sepsis, multi organ failure and death.

The ability to slide the NGT into the correct hole is like sinking a 20-foot putt; it takes a lot of practice and Sonya was way under par in the game of NGT placement.

"Go ahead and prep." I told Shana as I walked out to the sink with Angel.

By this time, Shana had completed the entire checklist except for the prepping and the time out. The former takes a minimum of 5 minutes and the latter 5 seconds. When she starts rubbing the skin with the sponges soaked in the light pink surgical soap, she glances at the wall clock and begins timing. For a full five minutes, she continually washes the skin with five separate sponges. She discards one every minute until all are gone and the clock verifies a five minute time span. While Shana preps, BJ and Jason stand by the back table, gowned and gloved, waiting on Angel and me. After sterilizing our hands and forearms, Angel and I enter the room. BJ and Jason gown and glove each of us; Shana completes her prep, and ties the back strings on our gowns and ask for a time out.

"Okay. Time out please." She announces as she steps back from us. We all stop and wait for her. Shana goes to her chart and reads out loud. "Georgia Anne Conway. Exploratory laparotomy and placement of central line for perforated viscus with peritonitis, sepsis, and dehydration. Permit signed by daughter, Patsy Conway, and is on the chart. Allergic to Sulfur. Received a gram of Invanz at 7:30pm and is now also getting a gram of Flagyl."

Angel, myself, Bj, Jason, and Sonya all echo together, " Agree." Informed consent, time out, prep, preoperative evaluation, resuscitation, and preparation were now all complete. We had been cleared for takeoff in OR room B. Georgia's abdomen, sterilized by alcohol and soap, smoothed by electric clippers, brightly lit by the dual LED ceiling mounted OR lights, enticed and captivated me with its hidden secrets, its warm, dark, moist caverns of multicolored treasures, its unseen, unilluminated recesses, fossas, quadrants, sacs, valves, beds, ligaments, flexures, curvatures, hilums, parts, segments, lumens, orifices, openings, lobes, surfaces, capsules, borders, layers, and lines. Somewhere in the world underneath the fleshy canopy of skin, fat, muscle, fascia, and peritoneum, lurked a dark angel from some paradise lost, some Charon, some evil serpent of deceit, destruction, and destitution, a harbinger of the abomination of desolation that the institution of medicine calls disease, pathology, infection, putrefaction, and death.

Unlike the great historical discoverers Polo, Zheng He, Dias, Vespucci, and Cabot, finders of wonders, lands, and people, my mission, each time I enter the abdominal cavity, is not to discover new organs or new anatomy, but uncover the source of sickness, the fountain of fever, the country of contamination, the producer of pestilence, or the manufacturer of malignancy; a game of search and repair. I am not just an explorer; I am also a disease defense builder, a rupture repairer, a restorer of ruined reserves, and a proletariat of pathology.

"What kind of incision are we doing?" asked Angel.

"Midline, above and below umbilicus." I answered. "We're starting now."

"We're starting now, "is the signal in my room for silence. No talking. No music. No noise except the background noise in the operating room like the regular, monotonous beeps of the heart rate monitor, the soft breezy swoosh of the respirator, the ding of the oxygen saturation monitor, the rushing of air from the compression boots, the background hum of the florescent ceiling lights, and the quiet rattle of papers and clicks of knobs from the anesthetist. In the midst of this relative silence, no voice is heard except my short, distinct hushed one word requests; "scalpel," "retractors," "cautery," "Adsons," Richardsons," "hemostat," 2-0chromic,".

Residency was different; no silence rule existed. Instead of requiring silence, the attending surgeons would request music.

Each attending would hand their CD folder to the circulating nurse before they scrubbed and gowned. The hospital CEOs, ever sensitive to surgeons' wants and desires and always desirous to promote a surgeons' loyalty, bought and placed in each OR a high end CD player and added loading and operating the CD player to the long list of circulating nurses' responsibilities.

Each attending had their own "music to cut by" and these unique songs reflected the personalities of the different attending surgeons but a few songs remained universally common among them; the songs "to close by".

The suturing of the incision is the universal sign of a finished job, the symbol of the successful completion of the tedious and difficult part of the operation, the gesture of relief, the foreshadowing of a fresh, hot cup of coffee in the doctor's lounge, and the divination of relaxation soon to follow. The surgeon's mood, emotions, and spirit during the closure is never better. The worry of complications, the tension of being error free, the anxiety of avoiding accidental injury to the patient, the concern of being too slow, are all gone and the ricochet effect is giddiness, exuberance, ebullience and the closing music reflects and mirrors these emotions. The most common songs for closing were the Stone's "can't get no satisfaction",, or Foreigner's "juke box hero", or Queen's "another one bites the dust", or the Eagle's "life in the fast lane".

This change in music from the soothing Mozart's piano concertos, Beethoven's symphonies, and Bach's baroque violin concertos to the body gyrating, foot taping, pelvic thrusting rock and roll transformed the somber mood of focused concentration to a party atmosphere of celebration and joy. Right in the middle of this closing music, the circulating nurse and techs began the instrument, sponge, and needle count. At the end of the count, the nurse would yell like a cheerleader "count correct" and the surgeon, assistant, and techs would quickly and boisterously respond in a high-pitched chorus "count correct".

The surgeon's musical authority, their right to choose, control, and command any music played in the OR, auditorily reminded everyone that the surgeon, and only the surgeon, mattered in any and all decisions even something as trivial as music selection; the surgeon was the king of a tiny kingdom completely enclosed in 600 square feet of tiled floor and walls. What the king wants or rather demands, the OR team quickly, silently, and reverently provides. The operating room is an autocratic monarchy and within its sterile confines there does not exist even the hint of democracy; no one votes because no vote is ever requested. The anesthetist, first assistant, circulating nurse, and OR techs never question the surgeon's authority; to question is equivalent to doubt and to doubt the surgeon is supreme heresy and blasphemy punishable by exile from the kingdom. The kingship is infallible, incontrovertible, and inerrant.

An example of this authoritative kingship occurred during residency. One of the most irascible, demanding, and fractious attending surgeons was the vascular surgeon Dr. Joseph Kayson. A tall, heavy man in his mid forties, with thick black eyebrows growing across his forehead in a bushy unibrow, he spoke with a deep Pennsylvania accented voice. He also had an irritating and annoying persistent peculiarity of speech; he ended every sentence in a lyrical tonal octave elevation like the end of the bob-white quail call-bob white! bob-white. Since he was a board certified vascular surgeon, trained at Emory University in Atlanta, he tolerated no one else's opinion about anything. His authority was absolute and his kingship was very much alive and well. All of the residents knew of his personality and we avoided operating with him as much as possible. If Dr. Kayson posted a complex vascular case, the chief resident, who always decided what resident would scrub with Dr. Kayson, invariably assigned anyone but him or her. One gloomy Monday, the chief resident assigned me, a third year resident, to Dr. Kayson's room for the entire day. I think she did this because I pissed her off the Friday before because I scrubbed and assisted with a lung resection without telling her. My failure to ask her permission and thereby give her first choice at operating in a big case was a punishable offense but I still feel her punishment was far too severe.

Dr. Kayson loved Mozart. It was, in my opinion, his only hint of humanity. Mozart's piano concerto no. 24 in C minor or his symphony no. 40 or, Dr. Kayson's favorite, Mozart's opera Don Giovanni , accompanied most of his surgeries. In Dr. Kayson's room, only two sounds were ever permitted, Mozart and Dr. Kayson's voice.

On that fateful Monday, the first case started at 7am. The patient, Robert Dickens, suffered from a multitude of self-inflicted diseases. He was a 66-year-old obese, chain smoking, diabetic with severe heart disease, lung disease, and peripheral vascular disease. His left common iliac artery(the main artery off the aorta that supplies blood flow to the left leg) was completely blocked but, miraculously, the right common iliac had minimal blockage which allowed blood to flow through some small pelvic arteries on the right side to the diseased left side below the blockage; it was enough to keep the left leg alive for a while but not enough to enable Mr. Dickens to walk more than ten feet without suffering severe left calf pain.

The operation, a fem-fem bypass, entailed cutting into the right groin artery (femoral artery), suturing a slender synthetic artery made of a man-made substance called Gortex, tunneling it under the skin at the bottom of the abdomen just above the base of the penis, cutting into the left groin artery and suturing the Gortex in place. Once completed, blood would flow across this Gortex from right to left and hopefully supply enough blood to the left leg without taking too much blood from the right; it worked a vast majority of the time, at least for a while but since Mr. Dickens chose not to lose weight, exercise, quit smoking, and take his medication as prescribed, it wouldn't last long and he would need a left leg amputation above the knee. Interestingly, an operation I would help perform two years later.

Don Giovanni was booming, Dr. Kayson was performing a Hillary Clinton joke soliloquy, and we had just finished suturing the Gortex into the good right groin artery. The Gortex tubing lay across the lower abdomen on top of and underneath sterile blue towels so only the ends were exposed.

"Okay resident (Dr. Kayson never called me or any other resident by name, we were just all the same nameless menial entities he had to tolerate like an animal trainer tolerates the cage door openers and whip cleaners and poop scoopers) time to switch." He moved over to the left groin and I moved over to the right groin. He had already opened the left groin artery so all that remained was suturing the Gortex into the left sided artery. Dr. Kayson began suturing; Don Giovanni had progressed to the middle of the aria, Dr. Kayson's favorite part.

"Excuse me Dr. Kayson?" asked Julie Hibbard, the circulating nurse.

"Nurse." He responded to her in the same manner as resident to us. "Do not talk. I'm in the middle of suturing this graft in place so whatever it is you need can just damn well wait."

"I don't think this can wait Dr. Kayson." She responded.

"Really nurse? Is the damn patient dying?"

"No sir."

"Is there a nuclear attack on the fricking country?"

"No sir."

"Then shut up."

"Yes sir." She answered. I looked at her and I saw some faint eye smile creases appear above her mask. She and I knew what Dr. Kayson didn't know but neither of us would violate his kingship.

Dr. Kayson finished the left groin artery anastomosis, unclamped the Gortex to allow blood to flow from the right to the left, and inspected both suture lines; both were perfect. No leakage of blood. Good pulses in both groin arteries and good pulses in both right and left feet; a complete and totally successful result.

"Alright resident. You can close." He announced as he backed away from the table and removed his gown and gloves. But just before he walked toward the door, I removed the blue towel. Dr. Kayson looked at the Gortex laying there on top of the skin; he had forgotten to tunnel it under the skin before he sutured the left side. Julie had attempted to tell him; and he now knew it.

"Should I get you another gown and gloves Dr. Kayson?" She asked snickering slightly.

"No. You can get the hell out of my room and get me another nurse in here."

CHAPTER 3

THE COLONOSCOPY

For several years, twice a week, I visited the Speedway, a small gas station in downtown Manchester, and bought a cup of dark roast black coffee. They used filtered water, Columbian coffee beans, and always made it fresh and since Starbucks did not and never will exist in Manchester, the Speedway's coffee ruled. Usually I paid 99 cents but occasionally Speedway would run a special and reduce the cost to 79 cents. Inside the store, the coffee counter spread along the wall across from the milk refrigerator, and consisted of six glass coffee pots, each labeled with a specific roast, and each sitting on separate warmers. After I poured the dark roast into a 16 oz. cup, on most mornings, Carolyn Kingston would check me out.

"Hey doc. How's it going?" She winked and smiled at me.

"Great Carolyn. Best day ever." I would respond. "How about you?"

"Blessed doc. Just blessed to be alive and to have a job."

This meet and greet with Carolyn continued for about two years before things changed; and they changed really fast. One Tuesday morning she came to my office.

"Well, looks like you get to serve me for a change uh doc?" She told me while sitting in my exam room.

"It will be a pleasure Carolyn. What's up with you?"

"Oh, something silly I guess but my doctor told me to come see you so here I am."

"Why did she send you?"

"Blood. Blood in my stools I guess. Anyway, she does this test of my stool and calls me and says she has found some cult blood. Whatever that is."

"I think she meant to say occult blood Carolyn. It's blood detectable by a chemical but not blood you can see."

"Oh. Well, anyway she says I need one of those scope things and asks me what doctor I waned to go see and I told her my coffee doctor of course " She smiles and winks at me.

"Any family history of colon cancer?"

"Nope. I don't remember any. My mother died of a heart attack and I never knew my dad."

"How old was your mom when she died?"

"Well let's see. She died about a year before I started working at the Speedway and I've been working there for six years so that means she died about seven years ago; I guess she was around 68. Yep. I think she was 68."

"How old are you Carolyn?"

"Now doc. Do I have to tell you? It ain't proper to ask a woman her age you know." She laughs and winks at the same time.

"Well, anything you tell me in this room is confidential and so I can't tell anyone else what you tell me."

"Oh yea. Don't you call that the Hypocritical oath?"

"Yeah. That's what we call it and it binds me to secrecy."

"Ok. I'm 39." She winks again.

"Thirty nine plus what?"

"Twenty."

"Ok."

After bantering for a while longer I finally get her scheduled for the colonoscopy. Colonoscopies are as common as a cold but they can be uncommonly difficult procedures. I once believed I was well trained in the technical aspects of them until I had been in practice for about a year.

I was leaving the hospital after completing a full day of colonoscopies when I met one of the local gastroenterologists leaving at the same time. We talked briefly about the day and she mentioned she had completed 12 colonoscopies for the day. I admitted I had performed 6. We went on our way but that really bothered me. How could she have finished twice as many scopes as me? I knew that there had to be a reason other than just patient variability. I decided to research colonoscopy techniques. I found an article, written by a surgeon in Opelika, Alabama, published in the American Surgeon, a well read and respected journal.

In this article, he detailed his technique. He would adjust the control knobs and advance and manipulate the scope at the same time. He did not use a tech to help with the scope except to hand him the instruments he needed to biopsy or remove polyps. This resulted in routinely reaching the cecum in less than five minutes! Unbelievable, I thought. This method was so different from the one I learned from my attending at the VA.

In residency, I performed all my colonoscopies at the VA hospital under the instruction of Dr. Miralles. Dr. Miralles used three people on every colonoscopy. He worked the controls that deflected the scope tip. By deflecting the scope tip up and down, and side to side, and by rotating the entire scope, we could see in 360 degrees; we could visualize the entire surface area of the colon.

Today, all colonoscopes are video. What is seen by the colonoscope is projected onto a high definition TV screen so the entire OR team can visualize exactly what the surgeon is seeing. In residency, however, the colonoscope was an eyepiece scope. The operator looked through the eyepiece like a telescope. No one else but the person looking through the eyepiece could see anything inside the colon. For Dr. Miralles to teach the resident, he attached to the eyepiece an extension called a teaching eyepiece. The extension cable was two feet long so the resident, standing beside Dr. Miralles, could see exactly what Dr. Miralles saw. The other end of the scope, the end inside the colon, had to be steadily advanced to the end of the five-foot long colon. The advancement of the scope, the difficult and tedious part of the procedure, the part that could and did lead to inadvertent perforations of the colon, was solely accomplished by an OR tech; an OR tech advancing, retreating, rotating, wiggling, and thrusting the thumb size black scope totally blind; they could not see anything. So, Dr.

Miralles, in his thick Spanish accent, yelled his instructions.

" Advance." He would yell and the tech would push the scope forward and continue to push forward until Dr. Miralles would yell again, " Stop. Oh my Joey. You have pushed too hard. You are too strong today. You ate some Wheaties Joey? You drink too much coffee Joey? Now, pull back. Pull back Joey. Stop. No. You pull back too much Joey. Dr. Edwards and me cannot see well because you have pushed too far into some poop and now our scope dirty Joey. You wash the scope Joey. Push the water down the scope. Now, we can see. Push Joey. Push a little more. No, no. Stop. Okay. Now pull back a little. I think I see a polyp. Stop Joey."

This continued for thirty to forty minutes until we finally reached the cecum (the beginning of the colon but the end of the colonoscopy). At the end of my five year residency, my number of completed colonoscopies met the requirements of the accreditation organization so the department of surgery chairman, Dr. William Bowman, signed my certificate making me board eligible and allowing me to obtain hospital privileges for colonoscopies. But, the Dr. Miralles way did have some weaknesses and some interesting problems.

In the VA hospital system, the majority of patients are male. A female patient at the VA is not just a minority but also a downright oddity. One day an oddity arrived at the endoscopy suite. Rebecca Holmes, a 35-year-old veteran of the navy, was admitted for bleeding from her rectum resulting in severe anemia that required a blood transfusion of four units. Dr. Miralles was consulted to perform the colonoscopy and I was the assigned second year resident.

Rebecca's gender clearly made Dr. Miralles nervous. He stuttered his introduction and continued to stutter through his explanation of the procedure for informed consent. We placed her on her left side, bent her knees up toward her abdomen, injected her with a narcotic and a benzodiazepine for sedation, and we exposed the area.

"Please turn the lights down Joey. We must have some

modesty. We must not show too much." Joey dimmed the lights.

"Now. Joey. I will advance the scope first because she is a girl. You stand back Joey. Give me the scope." Joey gave his end to Dr. Miralles and after a few seconds of awkward silence, Dr. Miralles finally said, " Okay Joey. It is in. Now you can advance. So, advance Joey. No. Stop. That is enough. Oh my. Oh oh oh my. You see Dr. Edwards? You see right?"

"Yes sir. I see. Uh, Dr. Miralles. I think...."

He interrupted me and excitedly proclaimed, " this is terrible. She so young. So so young. Terrible. Joey, get me the biopsy wire. We have to biopsy this cancer. It is big. It is completely obstructing the colon. How has she been able to poop? How? Hurry Joey. Get me the biopsy wire."

"Uh Dr. Miralles? I don't think you want to biopsy this." I said in a quiet tone.

"What? You okay. You drink enough coffee? You up late? You on call last night? You must be tired. Don't you see the large cancer?"Joey gave him the wire with the tiny biting biopsy jaws at the end and Dr. Miralles quickly advanced the wire down the scope channel but before he could reach the mass, I stopped him.

"Joey, turn on the lights. Dr. Miralles. Please look at your scope. You are not in the colon. You're in the vagina and you're about to biopsy what looks to me to be a perfectly normal cervix."

In my colonoscopies, the rule of absolute silence does not exist. Since most endoscopic procedures are not stressful, talking through the entire procedure is usually allowed. When I started advancing the scope on Carolyn, I continued talking with Johnny Jarvis and Cleo Sanders, the two techs, Wendy Lovins, the circulating nurse, and Bobby Monk, the anesthetist.

"Did I ever tell you guys the riddle of the two frozen people?" I asked. As I perform a colonoscopy, I usually call out the diagnoses as I encounter them so the circulating nurse can write them down in the chart. "Stage II internal hemorrhoids", I called out to Wendy. I continue to advance and I continued to talk.

"Uh no doc. I don't think you have." Answered Bobby.

"I told this to my youngest kids the other day and they never did get the answer. Well, this explorer finds these two perfectly preserved, frozen, naked bodies in a glacier in the Antarctica and after the team brings them up and the light shines on them, the explorer say, 'God almighty. This man is Adam and this woman is Eve'. Now, the question is, how did he know that? Oh Wendy, sigmoid diverticula scattered, not bleeding and not inflamed. Colonic diverticula are holes in the lining of the colon where the lining has punched out through the muscle layer and formed a weak, thin walled pouch on the outer surface of the colon. They exist in about 80% of the colons in America. They are caused by a fast food diet low in fiber. They never cause cancer, but can cause bleeding, infection, perforation, abscess, peritonitis, and death; but most of the time they don't cause any symptoms.

"Well I don't know doc." Answered Bobby. "You guys know the answer?"

"They had some fig leaves covering their privates." Offered Johnny.

"No. I told you they were completely naked."

"Oh yea. Well, they had tattoos with the name Adam and Eve." Johnny laughed.

"No. These are the original first man and woman." I answer.

"Oh we don't know doc. Go ahead and tell us." Responded Cleo.

"Everybody give up?" I ask. They all nodded their heads. "Holy moly. Wendy, large polyp. Sigmoid colon at 80 centimeters."

Flowing up from the light pink flat plain of colon cells, the normal mucosa, a purplish pink earthworm color tissue mass protruded upward into a volcano shaped ugliness. On its undulating top, an ulcerated crater of dead and dying cells oozed a magma of mucous, blood, and pus. The base spread horizontally for several centimeters before blending into the normal mucosa. The top of the ulcerated polyp stood six centimeters above the indistinct, blurred base; it was impossible to distinguish the end of normal colon cells and the start of the abnormal.

"Think you can get it all with the snare?" Asked BJ. I studied the mass for another few seconds.

"I think I can but I'll have to remove it in pieces. Okay. Lets set up for a polypectomy. Set the cautery to 20/20 and attach the suction trap."

Removing polyps (polypectomies) can be difficult if the polyps are large, ulcerated, wide based, or bleeding; like Carolyn's. Most colon polyps sprout from a thin, short stalk, bloom a 5mm tissue flower, retain a smooth, velvety, petal-like appearance, and are deceptively beautiful. I can easily loop my snare around their stalk, slide the loop down to its base, tighten it into a strangulating noose, torch it with electrical energy until it falls off leaving a charred bloodless ulcer, suction it into the colonoscope channel, irrigate it out into a filter trap, deposit it in a small jar of formaldehyde, and send it to the pathologist; the entire process takes less than five minutes. But not Carolyn's. Removing her polyp will be tedious, frustrating, and challenging.

Imagine a small, young, active mouse capering around a small cage furnished with an exercise wheel, food bowl, wooden chew block, hanging water bottle, and a plastic igloo house. You have to catch her and remove her from the cage. However, there are two restrictions. First, a wire mesh is welded across the top of the cage with mesh spaces barely large enough to pull the mouse's foot through. Secondly, you can only use a five foot straw sized metal tube with a loop of string dangling from the end. With this device only, you have to lasso the mouse's feet, tighten the loop until it strangulates and cuts through the tissue and then remove the entire mouse in tiny pieces small enough to pass through the mesh. That is slightly easier than removing Carolyn's entire polyp.

Removing the ulcerated volcanic top was the easy part; it was the base that worried me. Jason pushed the snare down the scope channel until the end emerged from the other end. He then opened the snare by squeezing a lever. The opened snare formed a wire loop suitable for lassoing the volcanic stalk. BJ held the scope still at the anus while I manipulated the lasso over the ulcerated crater and down the stalk until it rested against the large base.

"Close it." I yelled. Jason retracted the loop back until it tightened around the junction between the stalk and the broad base. I stepped on the cautery pedal and electrocuted the tissue. Smoke billowed up obscuring everything. Once the smoke cleared, the volcanic stalk and ulcerated top lay on its side, separated from the base, like a white oak hewed and felled. This severed portion was too large to remove from the colon by suctioning it down the narrow scope channel. Jason pulled the snare out of the scope and pushed another catheter down the scope and out into the lumen. This catheter did not have the wire loop snare but rather a small mesh net. I tightened the net around the downed portion, secured it tight against the end of the scope, and pulled the scope and the netted tissue out of the colon as a unit. I dropped it into the formaldehyde jar, cleaned the scope tip with saline and pushed it back to the 80-centimeter mark.

With the volcano stalk and crater gone, the base looked even more ominous. Instead of flat, it humped up from the normal tissue forming a homely, indistinct, sloping ledge; no clear delineated sharp shelf existed. The base was too flat to loop with the wire snare, too indistinct to be certain of its total removal, too low to remove without a high risk of cutting through the entire 3mm thick colon wall; it could not be removed with the scope. A flat polyp base 2 inches wide and 3 inches long remained and there was nothing I could do about it.

"Think you can get the rest?" Asked Jason. I photographed the polyp base and reluctantly admitted I couldn't safely remove it.

" What're going to do doc?" Asked BJ this time.

"I'm going to finish the colonoscopy and leave it."

"Do you think its cancer?" Asked Wendy.

I hate cancer. It looks ugly, and disgusting, and sinister; and it acts exactly the way it looks. It must be what hell looks like. Satan may be the loveliest angel ever to exist but what comes from him is revoltingly grotesque. Colon cancer, like most cancers, is a histological paradox, a cellular inconsistency, an absurdity in design. It attaches to healthy tissue with a violent tenacity only invasion could accomplish. This invasive adherence is the reason why removing cancer from the normal tissue, separating it and thus resecting it with margins of healthy tissue, in essence curing it, the ultimate goal of every surgeon, is often impossible; the cancer cells grow into, attach to, and become an alien part of the normal tissue. This is the first paradox; cancer becomes a cellular part of a normal organ and yet is totally different from the normal cells making it impossible to remove the cancer without removing the normal tissue as well; the cancer is thus not able to be resected; incurable because removing the cancer will kill the patient.

But there is a second paradox much more disturbing than the first. The second paradox is its monstrous, illogical, and vile immortality; the immortality of death. A cell is defined as cancerous if it has no function, no purpose, no service but to live and grow. All normal, healthy cells function to provide life for the body; lung cells diffuse oxygen, heart cells push blood, brains cells transmit chemical information, kidney cells absorb water, liver cells secrete bile, spleen cells purify blood, bone marrow cells manufacture blood, adrenal cells discharge epinephrine, skin cells sweat, hair cells grow, stomach cells absorb, and muscle cells move but cancer cells do nothing but replicate; they just survive while everything foreign to it dies. Cancer is both homicidal and suicidal.

When a kidney cell stops absorbing water and just starts replicating and growing, it's a kidney cancer. Cancer doesn't invade us like a bacteria or virus, making us sick from something outside of the body or from something we inhale or drink or eat. Some things in the environment do cause a normal cell to change into cancer but the cancer still originates within us; from our own body.

In the abdominal cavity, a kidney looks like a kidney, a spleen like a spleen, a liver like a liver. If I remove these organs and lay them, side by side, on the back table, and the OR techs rearrange them while I'm not looking and ask me to identify them, I could easily do it. However, if I remove a kidney cancer, a splenic cancer, and a liver cancer and lay them in a row and repeat the experiment, I could not tell the difference; the different cancers from different organs all look identical.

This bland, monotonous, indistinct appearance is the opposite of God's creative uniqueness. Remove order, structure, purpose, function, beauty, and color from any organ tissue and what you have left is cancerous tissue. God gives life its uniqueness, its uncommonness, its singularity, its beauty. The inimitableness of life is from God; the oneness, the sameness, the boringly uninteresting, the purposeless, the blandness, the structure less, and the colorless, are all from Satan.

Skin cancer obliterates the unique fingerprint, changing its uniqueness into a undecipherable blob. Breast cancer exterminates the breast's sexual beauty and renders it a mutilated lump. Lung cancer expunges the energizing stimulus of oxygen and breeds a mucous and blood expectoration. Colon cancer transforms the easy natural excretion of waste into a blocked bowel of sewage and putrefaction. Chaos, disorder, and death always follow Satan and his most devastating prodigy.

"Yes. It sure looks like cancer."

As I leave the room, I can only think about how I'm going to tell her. Medical school and residency never taught me the best and least frightening way to say, 'you have cancer'. Before I leave, Bobbie Monk called out to me.

"Hey doc. What's the answer? To the riddle. How did the explorer know it was Adam and Eve?"

I looked back at him and everyone waited to hear my answer. Until then I had completely forgotten about the riddle.

"Remember that Adam and Eve were unique. They were the first. They didn't have belly buttons. They were created, not born."

CHAPTER 4

THE ABDOMEN

In this abdomen, in this peritoneal cavity, in this dark, moist, warm, body cave, somewhere, is a hole. I had to find it. I had to find it fast. I had to find it, close it, repair or resect the organ it was in, wash out the leaked fluid, blood, stool, acid, food, and bacteria with liters of warm saline and then close the peritoneum, fascia, muscle, subcutaneous tissue, and skin. The longer it took to do this, the greater the chance of complications and death. The first few hours were the most critical and Georgia had already been perforated for at least six hours. I needed no phone calls, no pagers, no music, no chitchat, no riddles, no jokes, no distractions.

"Scalpel."

BJ held it, pinched between his right thumb and second finger, on the top, with the cutting edge facing down.

"Scalpel." He repeated before he passed it. His echo response was both an acknowledgement and a warning; he understood what I wanted and he was telling the rest of the team to be careful and pay attention; he's passing a scalpel across the patient and past them.

I took it and pressed the cold, hard, surgical steel between my thumb and second finger and rested it on my third. To steady and guide my hand, I lightly leaned the third, fourth and fifth fingertips against Georgia's orange prepped skin. I pushed the scalpel edge against the skin and dragged it backwards toward me. Trailing behind the slicing scalpel, marking the path, appeared a thin line of blood. After seven inches, I announced the warning again, "scalpel back."

"Cautery." Angel handed me the pencil sized plastic disposable cautery device, wiped the blood off the incision with the lap sponge, and held the suction over it while I burnt the bleeding skin vessels. With each zap of the cautery, smoke billowed up from the burning tissue and blood, a pungent burning human flesh smell rose higher and more powerfully than the resultant smoke. The odor, although not unpleasant, was distinct. I cauterized and Angel worked the suction. No one wanted to smell it or inhale it.

We stopped all the skin bleeding, pulled the skin edges apart, and looked at the bottom of the furrowed incision. At the bottom was the brownish-yellow subcutaneous fat. In this layer, just under the skin, only a few veins coursed. A nuisance layer of tissue with little use other than stored calories. It harbored no major structures, produced no major hormones, offered little defense except against extreme cold, and secreted only liquefied fat into the blood stream. I cut though this butter like tissue easily with the cautery. In some, this layer is many inches thick but in Georgia, it was barely two inches before I saw the fascia.

In the mid abdomen, the rectus muscle quivered and jerked between two layers of fascia; a top and a bottom layer. Underneath the top layer, the beefy muscle, the six-pack muscle, stretched vertically from the end of the breastbone to the top of the pelvis. Georgia's rectus muscle, sandwiched between the fascial sheaves, like most women and men of similar age, presented no sensuous bulge, no envious sharp outline, no thick muscle ribbons. In Georgia, the muscles flattened into thin separated wafers, divorced from their bed of youthful nestle, residing inches apart, allowing the intrusion of the bulging underneath fascia to rise up between them.

Both layers of the white, smooth, tough fascia, regardless of how weak they become, protects and defends the vital abdominal cavity contents far better than the thick skin, oily subcutaneous fat, and watery muscle. Underneath its one millimeter thickness, rubbing and sliding against its underside, is the one cell thick peritoneum, a membrane thinner than cellophane, rich with nerves, lymphatic channels, and immune cells and it is continuously lubricating the muscle walls and vital organs in the abdominal cavity. The peritoneum is the body's watchdog, alarm system, Security Company. Violate its surface with even one cubic centimeter of air and it will send pain signals to the brain. Rub it with a gloved finger in an awake patient and they will moan with pain. One drop of gastric acid on it will force a grown man to scream in pain.

The fascia shields, secures, and safeguards the abdominal cavity structures: the pulsating blood vessels, filtering spleen, bilious liver, acidic stomach, enzymatic pancreas, excreting kidneys, absorbing intestines, and malodorous colon. Opening the fascia and peritoneum violates the sanctified inner chamber, the holiest of holies, the sepulcher of life. But I can only find the offending hole, the life threatening damage, the contamination by violently cutting into and through it. But cutting into the fascia is very risky. Cut one millimeter too deep and the pink, writhing coils and loops of intestine will be cut as well and then not only has my presence violated the sanctity and sterility of the inner chamber but now I have desecrated the ark, the lamp stand, the pedestal, the very seat of life.

In the rush to find and repair the life threatening disease, an overzealous, clumsy, fumbling abdominal cavity entrance will unintentionally injure the intestines magnifying the already severe damage. Unfortunately, this inadvertent injury, by a surgeon or a surgeons' assistant, happens enough to have a medical name; iatrogenic. An iatrogenic injury can be as insignificant as a small cut in an inconsequential vein or artery requiring a simple suture or as severe as a long gash in the unforgiving bacteria harboring large intestine requiring the removal of some colon and forming a colostomy by suturing some of the colon to the skin.

To prevent this iatrogenic injury, I will pinch and elevate, between two hemostats, a small segment of fascia. By elevating or stretching the fascia, I can create a safe space of a centimeter between the intestines and the underside of the fascia. To accomplish this, the patient must be paralyzed. Muscle paralysis is accomplished with a specific drug the anesthetist gives in the IV.

"Is she paralyzed?" I asked Sonya as I stared at the fascia.

"Let me check. "She grabbed a small square shaped device , the size of a hand warmer, called a nerve stimulator. The battery-operated device has two short thick metal poles, separated by two inches, sticking out like antenna. She pressed them against Georgia' left neck and pushed the energy button. A low voltage electric current surged into the skin, passed down through the subcutaneous fat and entered the platysma, a thin, superficial enveloping neck muscle. The neck muscle didn't move. If the amount of paralyzing drug Sonya had injected in Georgia was too low, the platysma would twitch and jerk in a spasmodic reaction to the nerve stimulator. But if the drug level was high, the platysma would not respond to the electrical current.

"No twitch doc. We're good".

"Curved hemostat."

"Curved hemostat doc." BJ echoed. He grasped the closed end of the instrument, laterally rotated his right wrist and then quickly and decisively flipped his wrist back and slapped the handle end into my outstretched and open right palm. Like a strong handshake, it was firm, forceful, and formidable; and it felt good. When it hit my palm, my hand reflexively closed, my thumb and second finger slipped into the handle holes, and opened the hinged end. The entire instrument passing maneuver, from my request, through the slap and transference, to my automatic opening, took two seconds.

The passing of surgical instruments from scrub tech to surgeon is older than the gowns, masks, and gloves. Before Halstead, Billroth, Cushing, DeBakey, and Cooley, before Morris's sleeping gas, before Larrey's military surgeries under Napoleon, before Carrel's artery suturing, before Blalock's heart tetralogy, operating rooms resounded with the smack of instruments from bare hands to bare hands.

It is the auditory symbol of surgery itself and the very nature and essence of surgeons themselves. Surgery demands decisiveness, willful and forceful resolve, and a determined and persistent attitude. In the operating room, a weak wimpy handshake, a shy diffident personality, a contemplative meditative character, is foreign to a surgeon and a slow, weak instrument pass is just as alien and as intolerable. Quick, confident, decisive, unhesitatingly forceful are the attributes of a surgeon. One famous surgeon said it this way, 'if you must cut, and you must, then cut boldly.'

The diseases a surgeon faces are not wimpy, weak, or wavering. To defeat them, to cure them, to extricate them, or to ameliorate them, a greater force than the power of disease or injury must be used. To have the best chance of defeating your enemy, you must know your enemy well. Surgery is like that. It is a battle against formidable and powerful forces. Disease is like a soldier fighting under the generalship of death. Failure to defeat the disease always leads to death. The victory over disease is, of course, a temporary celebration. Ultimate defeat to death is inevitable, immutable, and inexorable. But surgeons fight on anyway. The Greeks defined heroism in a unique manner. Unlike today, when we equate heroism as lack of cowardice and fear, or a presence of great courage and self-sacrifice, the Greeks defined it as an attitude. If you know you will lose, if you know you have no hope of winning and yet you fight anyway, then you are a hero. So, using this definition of heroism, all of us who daily go to work, encourage and uplift our children, show kindness and forgiveness, demonstrate compassion, nonjudgmentally engage in human relationships, cry when our friends cry and laugh when they laugh, send gifts to our enemies, and respond to every human need, are heroes.

Timidity in the operating room, by any team member, affronts the nature of surgery, insults the surgeon, discredits the mission of surgery, weakens the OR teams' resolve, and lowers the morale. It is a serious offense and results in ostracism from the operating room. Surgeons do not tolerate weakness by any OR team member; including themselves. Often, the surgeon is a different person in the OR than outside.

In the operating room, a surgeon is deliberate, willful, calculated, and resolved. Outside the operating room, they can have an exact opposite personality. One of my residency professors was Dr. Joyce Mclemore. A tall, thin, gray-haired, middle-aged, spinster with horn rim glasses, a string of pearls around her thin chicken-like neck and a wardrobe consisting of only ankle length, slightly different shades of blue, thin, high neck collared, cotton dresses. Like her attire and physical appearance, she was, outside the OR, a reticent, unimposing, meek mouse of a woman. She didn't look like a surgeon, didn't dress like one, didn't speak like one. She acted more like an old first grade school teacher. However, in the OR, she was a terror.

As soon as she put on the sterile, green, surgical garments, she became not only a monarch, but also a priest in full vestments celebrating the Eucharist, a preacher pounding the pulpit, a sweating, red-faced hollering cleric reveling in his temporary moment of significance, his uninterrupted period of unflinching attention from a group of otherwise self-motivated, self-indulgent practitioners of iniquity.

In residency, all of us residents had derogatory, degrading, and demeaning nicknames given to us as interns. Sometimes the chief resident bestowed it on us but more often, the attending surgeons picked them out. The criteria used to pick the name always remained a mystery but certain trends did emerge. One of the second year residents, Mark Glascock, a short, obese, balding man from South Carolina, had an annoying and unique habit of licking his lips several times during any conversation that lasted longer than a few sentences; a kind of visual stutter. The chief resident dubbed him "Flick". During hospital rounds, Joan Westerfield, the chief surgeon, a thin, flat chested, cachectic wisp of a woman from San Antonio, loved to have him on her team; she apparently loved his nickname even though she was not the chief resident who named him.

"Hey Flick." She would yell out at the first patient bedside. "Hey Flick, present this man's case for us". She smiled at him and the rest of the medical students while the interns, including me, just looked at the floor hoping she wouldn't call on us and us.

Then Flick would start rattling off the information. "Sixty-nine year old Caucasian (lick, lick, lick) male presented with a three day history (lick, lick, lick) of diffuse abdominal pain (lick, lick, lick) associated with nausea, vomiting, anorexia (lick, lick, lick) and fever..." She would laugh at him the whole time and finally she would stop him. "That's enough Flick. I can't laugh anymore. My sides are killing me." I never did learn what her nickname was since chief residents were immune from any name other than doctor sir, or doctor ma'am. But I came up with one I thought was good, even though I never used it, "stick girl."

My first chief resident, Rafael Gaines, gave my nickname to me. He was a former college basketball player from Florida. He stood six feet six inches, wore size 15 shoes, had hands bigger than a catcher's mitt, and his wrists' circumference was longer than my biceps. But despite his size, he talked with the most girlish voice I have ever heard from a man. I did learn his nickname, although, again, I never used it; "squeaker".

I spent the first month of my intern year assigned to the urologist service under the attending Dr. Reyansh Agarwals (Dr. A for short). Dr. A, because he was a VA urologist, had a very busy practice. But since most of his operations were endoscopic partial prostate resection for difficulty urinating, and since those operations would always be performed by a urologist and not a general surgeon, and since it was an operation not requiring my assistance, I had enough free time to work in the VA emergency room suturing lacerations. I spent several hours a day suturing any and all lacerations. The ER physicians loved me because I made it possible for them to sleep longer and work less for the same amount of pay because the VA paid them by the hour, not by the patient encounter. It didn't take Rafael long to discover where I was each afternoon.

"Well Dr. Dana Edwards. I see you have spent another whole afternoon in the ER. It seems that is all you like to do. Stay in the ER. So I think a good name for you is Daner. So Daner, when you finish today in the ER, I need you to go help in ICU put in some central lines." The nickname stuck.

"Curved hemostat to me." Angel called immediately after I asked.

"Curved hemostat Angel." BJ passed it to her and she mimicked my prior movements, spread the hemostat open, and hovered the open jaws over the exposed fascia. Angel is my surgical first assistant, my business partner, and my wife. After we married, the medical group who employed us, instituted a rule prohibiting spouses from working in the same department. Because of that, we immediately moved to Manchester, opened our own surgical practice, and started operating together on every surgical case. All that happened over 20 years and six children ago.

The first assistant's job is to make every surgeon look better. The best first assistants are the ones who anticipate, from experience, what the surgeon's next move will be. By knowing the surgeons' routine, the first assistant is always ready before the surgeon needs to ask for an instrument, a sponge, a suture, cautery, or suction. The operation proceeds smoothly, uninterruptedly, without stops and starts, and without any wasted movements or wasted time. If Angel is not available to help me during an operation, then I have to spend time instructing the assistant on everything I need them to do.

I stop, tell them to get a similar pair of DeBakey pickups, tell them to grasp the tissue opposite me, tell them to please suction out the blood, tell them to cauterize a blood vessel I have clamped in my hemostat, tell them to cut the suture, tell them to irrigate the incision, tell them to pull harder on the retractor, tell them what size retractor to use, tell them to adjust the lights. An operation is a series of moves that must proceed in a prescribed logical manner and after operating with me for several years, Angel had memorized the moves so she knew all of the steps, in their order, for every operation. The savings in time is enormous and can reduce a typical two hour operation into a one hour. With a good first assistant, I can increase the number of operations performed in eight hours by 30% and with a great first assistant, like Angel, I can easily double the number of surgeries per day.

I placed my hemostat on the fascia and whispered, " Grab." Angel placed hers a half inch opposite mine.

"New scalpel, 15."

"New scalpel, 15, open." Repeated BJ. "Lift." Angel and I lifted our hemostats upward, stretching and elevating the attached paralyzed muscle fascia two centimeters away from the abdominal cavity structures resting in the dark just underneath. I pressed the scalpel against the fascia between our hemostats and cut a 3mm hole. We stared into the dark underneath. Angel adjusted the light and illuminated the cavity. The light pink glistening surface of a loop of serpentine bowel reflected the bright light.

"Metzenbaums." I whispered.

"Metzenbaums." Repeated BJ. He slapped the slightly curved seven-inch long scissors into my right hand. I slid the opened jaws into the hole, slowly cut up toward the lower chest until I had safely opened a fascial rent long enough and wide enough to admit my hand. For the first time in 40 years, Georgia's abdominal cavity lay open, unconcealed, naked to the atmosphere and lights of an operating room. Finally, her abdominal cavity was exposed to my sight, my touch, my hearing, and my smell. I looked across at Angel but she was already looking at me with her big, blue eyes.

"Do you smell it?" I asked impatiently. She shook her head.

"Dana, what are we going to do?"

CHAPTER 5

THE SURPRISE

Pathologists are funny people in an unfunny profession. How could a person be a pathologist without having a somewhat unusual personality? They work alone, in a small office, looking down a microscope at slides fixed and stained with chemicals and preservatives, counting cellular features like an accountant counting pay stubs. They tally up the different mitotic figures, nuclear bodies, replicating cells, presence or absence of certain chemical stains, height of cells, width of cells, number of cells, and color of cytoplasm. They use all these 'facts' to make a final and definitive diagnosis; this person has well differentiated breast adenocarcinoma, this person has poorly differentiated prostate cancer, this person has premalignant changes etc. Their professional excitement, their adrenaline rush, is not exploring the living anesthetized human body in the operating room. Their excitement is listing the facts displayed in the microscopic world of dead tissue, finding all the abnormalities and then making a diagnosis. As is known, from countless autopsies, pathologist always knows the correct diagnosis, just too late to help the patient.

To a pathologist, the titillation in finding malignant cells in a tissue biopsy is similar to the hysteria Howard Carter experienced when he discovered the steps to the lost tomb of Tutankhamen. So when the pathologist called me, I knew it would be bad news. Good news never motivates a pathologist.

"Hey Dana. This is Joyce Nefew. How are you?" She sounded far too happy.

"Hey Joyce. I'm fine. You have some news for me?"

"Yeah. The polyp on your patient Carolyn Kingston. I just

finished signing it out. You'll get the written report tomorrow for her chart but I thought I better give you a heads up."

"Bad news I guess?"

"Well. Yeah. I'm signing it out as poorly differentiated invasive adenocarcinoma. The margins are not clear and there is some vascular and lymphatic invasion as well. I guess you'll have to do a resection?"

"I think so Joyce. The polyp base is just too broad and flat to be safely removed with the scope."

"Well, sorry to give you bad news. I hope she does well. I'll be looking for the colon and lymph nodes later. Hey, have a good day."

"You too Joyce. And thanks again."

Pathologists are funny for another and more interesting reason; they all want a disease named after them. It's easy to understand this eponymic ambition in an astronomer or early world explorer or astrophysicist or chemist but not in a pathologist. Personally, I don't want my name to be inextricably linked to a human malady. But pathologists constantly work with the hope they will be the first to discover a new disease, a new pathological diagnosis, a new complex syndrome. Dozens of eponymic diseases exist and every pathologist wishes one of them had been named after them instead of Drs. Cruveilhier, Paget, Hansen, Cushing, Hashimoto, Whipple, Bright, and Zenker.

Pathologists slice up preserved human tissue, place those pieces on dozens of labeled microscope slides, add a variety of chemical dyes, wait a prescribed number of hours for the tissue to "fix", and then spend hours hunched over a double eyepiece microscope detailing and comparing their findings against a mental list of hundreds of diseases until their they can make a match. Their work is tedious, long, and isolated. They work alone. Pathologists don't work in brightly illuminated, sterile, stainless steel operating rooms surrounded by a team of professionals just waiting for directions. Nor do they work in the chaotic, fast paced emergency room or even in a medical clinic populated with constantly rotating patients with the same mundane chronic complaints.

Pathologists work in small, windowless, dim, sparsely furnished offices. They need little in support and they receive little. A sturdy table, comfortable swivel chair, a computer and an assistant to help process human tissue is all they need. They don't need nurses, respiratory therapists, anesthetists, operating room techs, first assistants, pharmacists, information specialists, case manager, occupational therapists, physical therapists, admission clerks, pulmonologists, cardiologists, or gastroenterologists; occasionally, they may need a phone so they can excitedly call a surgeon.

After I spoke with Joyce, I moved Carolyn's appointment up to the next day instead of the usual two weeks. She came alone. Divorced, grown children, dead parents, siblings living away, all explained Carolyn's solitude. She sat in the examining room chair as I entered and, as usual, she smiled when she saw me.

"Good morning Carolyn."

"Hey doc. How are you? "In all the years I bought coffee from her, she never once addressed me by my first name or by the more formal Dr. Edwards; it was always doc.

"I'm fine, How are you?"

"Well, I guess you'll tell me that doc." She looked at me and her green eyes revealed how worried she was. "I guess you don't call patients in early to tell-'em good news. Am I right?"

I looked at her sitting there alone. She wore a long sleeve light blue blouse tucked into a beige loose skirt. She displayed a long necklace of pearls, pearl earrings, and dark brown ankle high boots. She kept her ringless hands folded in her lap holding a small dark blue purse. She looked like she had dinner plans with some friends but they had failed to arrive.

"Carolyn, I never really know the best way to begin this conversation. I guess the best way is to just tell you the bad news first and go from there." I cleared my voice and waited for her response but she stayed silent.

"Carolyn, you have colon cancer." She sighed but otherwise said nothing.

"Well that's the bad news."

"Is there any good news Doc?" She was not smiling anymore.

"Well, yes. This appears to be early stage cancer so you have a great chance of cure." I tried to sound excited. "Of course the cure will begin with a colon resection."

"Yeah. I thought I'd have cancer. Something told me I'd have something bad. Anyway, I'm ready doc. Just tell me what we need to do to fix this. And please tell me you're the one to do my surgery. I'm just not going anywhere else."

"Okay Carolyn. I'm the one but I have to discuss options with you."

"You mean I have options?"

"Well, you don't have any other good options but legally I have to tell you what they are. You always have the legal right to do nothing. Of course if you don't have surgery then the cancer will continue to grow."

"What would happen to me if I didn't have surgery and I just let things happen? You know what they say about surgery and cancer? Once you operate and expose the cancer to the air then it'll grow fast and I'll be dead in a month." She spoke sincerely.

"I've heard that for years too Carolyn but you know it's just a wives tale. I think it came from cases when the surgeon opened up an abdomen and found extensive metastatic cancer and had to close the abdomen without being able to do anything to help. A surprise. Then when the patient died a month later a few ignorant people said the exposure to air accelerated the cancer growth causing the patient to die quickly. But, Carolyn, there is no evidence of any such surprise for you. Your cancer should be in a very early stage. It's even possible that surgery will cure you and you won't even need chemo."

"You still didn't answer my question doc."

"Oh. I forgot. Okay, if you don't have surgery, the cancer will continue to grow to the point it will block the colon causing a bowel obstruction. This obstruction will cause continuous nausea, vomiting, distention, severe pain, dehydration, kidney failure, colon perforation, peritonitis, sepsis, and death."

"Well. I guess you're pretty blunt aren't you doc?"

"Yeah. I am. You want to know the truth and you deserve to know all of it. But here is your second option. I take you to surgery, I do another colonoscopy while you're asleep, I find the cancer and mark the area with a dye called methylene blue so I can be sure what part of your colon I need to remove. Then I open your abdomen with a low midline incision running from your pelvic bone to your belly button. The cancer is located in the middle of your left colon so I'll remove about 6 inches of it and then rejoin the ends so you will not have a colostomy. The surgery will take about 2 hours, you'll wake up in recovery room and then you'll be transferred to ICU for about three days so we can use an epidural pump to keep your pain to a very low level. You'll stay in the hospital until your bowels start working again and you're eating well. That will take about six to seven days. You'll go home with a few pain pills and will be sore for about two weeks. After the pathologist examines the specimen, she'll be able to stage your cancer. But I still believe it will be an early and very curable state. While I'm inside your abdomen, I'll look at your liver as well and if I see anything abnormal I'll biopsy it. Once you have totally healed, I'll send you to a cancer specialist to determine if you would benefit from chemo or radiation treatment." I stopped and looked at her. She hadn't moved but tears were now trickling down her face. I gave her the tissue box.

"Any questions so far?"

"Just one. When can you do it?"

Mondays are my day. On Mondays, the hospital allows me to use two operating rooms simultaneously. I have two operating room teams, two anesthetists, two circulating nurses, and four OR techs plus Angel. The hospital CEO, Darlene Scofield, met with me several years ago and asked what she could do to increase the number of surgeries I perform weekly; I told her to give me full and sole control of the OR on Mondays. Don't allow any other surgeon to schedule any elective cases from 8am to 3pm and I could do twenty surgeries every Monday. Surprisingly, she agreed.

Since then, she has kept her promise and I have consistently delivered on mine.

On the Monday of Carolyn's surgery, I think the weather was cold, rainy, and windy. At least I do remember the weather was not pleasant.

In the holding area, I met her few relatives for the first time. I asked if Carolyn or any family member had a question; no one asked anything other than one older lady asked me to take good care of Carolyn. Nearly every major operation I perform has one family member present who will ask me to take good care of their family member. I realize it's their only way of verbally showing love and concern in a situation where they have no input, no control, and no authority. It's similar to flying in a commercial airplane; you buckle up, lean back, and then realize that your life, your existence in this world, is now in the hands of some stranger that you have never met or seen or talked with; a stranger who's qualifications as a pilot you know nothing about and who's personal life you know even less about. You wonder about their health, their age, their risk of a heart attack. You speculate about their drinking habits, their possible diabetes and absence of blood sugar monitoring, their compliance with seizure medications, if the airlines even allow pilots with seizure disorders to fly. Then you wonder if they are experienced in flying this particular type of aircraft and if they have ever flown this route before and have they ever had to deal with an inflight emergency. When a surgeon takes you or your family member back to surgery, I imagine similar doubts and fears.

"Will you pray for me Dr. Edwards?" For the first time she was formal. She looked at me and smiled her old familiar smile.

"Sure Carolyn. I'd love to." I placed both hands on her right shoulder and the family laid their hands on her and on me. I prayed my gospel of John prayer.

"Thanks Dr. Edwards." Carolyn squeezed my hand and the family all said amen.

One of the family members looked at me and said the one thing I hate, the one comment which I have always found disturbing and the one phrase I try my best to avoid by leaving before anyone can say it but today, Carolyn held my hand a little too long.

"Hey Dr. Edwards, thanks for a great prayer and good luck."

Good luck. Wow. What a revealing two-word phrase. Good luck. We just finished praying, we just gave God all the glory and praise, we just completed our verbal confirmation of His love and care, we just acknowledged that all healing is from Him, we just openly and publicly established the presence of the everlasting eternal God and our complete trust in Him, and then, barely one second later, we shove it all away and say we only believe in chance. We trust nothing but fortune. Why don't we just flip a coin? Heads and Carolyn will survive this major operation and tails, well; we'll go ahead and order the flowers. Oh, and lets do another coin toss for the cure of the cancer. Heads and Carolyn you will be totally healed but tails and we'll go ahead and get the hospital bed ready for your long, painful, miserable life waiting for you during the few months you have left to live.

Bob Monk intubated her, Wendy Lovings, the circulating nurse, placed a bladder catheter to drain her urine, the techs, Johnny Jarvis and Cleo Sanders, lifted her legs over the stirrups and tightened each leg strap, Bob lowered the half of the table below Carolyn's buttocks, Wendy prepped her abdomen with an antiseptic soap and prepped her genitalia and anus with an iodine based prep and Angel, Cleo, and Johnny draped her sterile abdomen and clean vagina and anus with two separate drapes; this allowed easy access to her rectum for the colonoscopy.

"Are we ready to start Bob?" He peeped over the sterile drapes and nodded. "Okay, Johnny, break out and help with the colonoscope. Angel, you can go ahead and numb the incision site. Bob, did you get the epidural in?" He peeped again and nodded.

"Great. Wendy, while I'm doing the colonoscopy, call up to ICU and make sure we have a bed. Johnny? Do you have the methylene blue and the endoscopic needle?"

"Yes sir doc. I have both on the scope tray."

"Okay. I'm starting now." Everyone looked at the clock and

Wendy wrote the time, 1:15pm.

"Johnny, go ahead and draw up ten milliliters of the dye and have it ready. Cleo, make sure we have two 15 scalpels. Angel, you finished numbing yet?"

"Of course."

I pushed the colonoscope into her rectum. " Wendy, did she get her antibiotics?"

"Running now Doc."

"Great. Johnny, the suction isn't working."

"I'll check doc."

"I got it Johnny." Said Wendy. She went over to the suction canister and checked the connections. "It's the connection to the canister. It should work now."

"Yep. It does. Thanks Wendy."

"I'm at 40. Johnny, go ahead and lets put the injection needle down but don't connect the dye syringe yet. You know what a mess that stuff can make if it leaks out."

"Okay doc. Here's the needle." He handed me the six foot long cable with the small injection needle safely pulled inside the tip to avoid injury when pushing it out the end of the scope.

"Okay. I'm at 60. It won't be long now."

"Oh, I forgot to ask doc. You want an NG tube(a plastic tube passed down the nose and into the stomach to prevent post-operative nausea and vomiting)?" Bob asked as he peered over the drapes.

"No. I don't think so Bob. We'll just wait on that but I don't need one now. Okay. I'm at 80."

At 1:20pm, I had passed the colonoscope to the location of the cancer. All I had to do was visualize it, push the endoscopic injection needle underneath it, inject the blue dye, and remove the colonoscope. The entire dye marking procedure takes me less than one minute. The sterile dye suffuses out into the sub mucosal tissue, leaks into the lymphatic channels, lodges in the surrounding lymph nodes, and within five minutes wraps the colon at the injection site with a three inch wide royal blue blanket. The stain transforms a difficult to feel cancer into a visual blue splotch in a sea of pinks, reds, yellows, and purples.

"I'm at 90." I look up at Angel and she looks back quizzically.

The exact location of a colon lesion, as measured during a colonoscopy, is accurate with a 20 cm margin of error. When a colonoscope is pushed along the colon lumen, the colon is not static, not paralyzed, not immobile; it moves like any other viable part of the intestine. Therefore, the length of colonoscope inside the colon is either shorter or longer than centimeter markers on the side of the colonoscope. It is what endoscopists call a telescope effect. So I pushed on.

"I'm at 100cm." I look at Angel again. She's still looking at me.

Surgeons always fear the possibility of missing a potentially life threatening disease either because of human error or technical failure. It is a real fear because it happens despite our greatest effort to prevent it. I saw it in residency and I have experienced it in practice. In a colonoscopy, if a known lesion is not where you thought it was, you simply keep looking; I kept looking.

"I'm at 110cm." The colon lining, the mucosa, looked pink, smooth, shiny, moist, normal. I pushed on.

"I'm at 120cm." Now for the first time I started to worry. Where was it? I saw it there less than 2 weeks ago. I partially removed it. I photographed the large, raised, base of cancer left behind. I talked with the pathologist personally to confirm the aggressive nature of the cancer. But I couldn't find it. I didn't look at Angel anymore.

At this point, I resorted to a complete relook colonoscopy. I went back to the cecum and then slowly, methodically, and desperately reevaluated the colon mucosa one centimeter at a time. I came all the way back to the rectum but still saw no lesion of any kind, size, or shape.

"What are you going to do Dana?" Angel looked at me after she asked the worst question she could ever ask me.

"I'm going to look again." I advanced all the way again to

the cecum and repeated the entire procedure again. But this time, starting at the 110 cm mark and continuing to the 60cm mark, I performed small blind biopsies of the mucosa. I still could not see anything abnormal but I thought maybe some unexpected swelling hid the lesion underneath the lining. After I finished, I removed the colonoscope. I stood there looking at the wall for a few seconds. Finally, I looked at Angel; she was crying.

No-one spoke. They all looked at me. I knew the truth. They all knew the truth as well. Everyone in that room had been in the room two weeks ago. Everyone had seen the polyp, the partial removal, the remaining ugly, large, raised, spreading base at 80 cm. There was no need to talk.

"We are done." I said and I walked out and went to the doctor's locker room. I sat on the small couch and looked at the ceiling. I reminded myself that cancers do not just go away. Without treatment, they don't melt or dissolve or die. They grow, not regress. They enlarge, not shrink. They expand, not shrivel. But the cancer that was there two weeks ago, had disappeared. But how? What really happened?

For me, I knew the answer. And I knew that soon, in fact just as soon as I walked out into the waiting room and explained to the family what happened, many people would know the truth; but for now, in the tiny locker room, sitting alone, I could only do what Angel had done. I cried like a silly baby.

CHAPTER 6

THE GHOST

The human abdominal cavity smells; it's a distinct smell, unlike anything else, and is the same regardless of race, age, or gender. If it could be bottled and then opened during a dinner party of prime rib, potatoes au gratin, broiled asparagus, and Caesar salad, I would, with one sniff, search the room for the unfortunate guest with the abdominal stab wound. The smell is subtle, not overwhelming; its distinctiveness, not it's strength, makes it so noticeable.

Place a row of freshly blooming flowers on a table, blindfold me, lead me by each flower and ask me to identify each one by its unique fragrance and I wouldn't properly identify any. But, if you set a newly opened bottle of abdominal cavity in the middle of all these fragrant inflorescences, I would tear the blindfold off and frantically search for the gravely injured person lying somewhere underneath the table.

The smell is difficult to describe since it isn't similar to many aromas. It's mildly pungent, like a raw cut of rib eye at room temperature. It's also rather disturbing; it is not pleasant. It's not fruity or woody or lemony, sweet, or sour. It's slightly sickening but only barely. It has none of the overwhelming, nauseating, malodorous aroma of feces, vomit, rotting meat, or bacterial laden pus.

If I could drink it, it would be like a nice steel barrel matured California Chardonnay, low acidity, moderately sweet, and very low in tannins.

Describing the smell of the human abdominal cavity is like trying to describe the emanation coming from an unblemished new born lamb roasting over an open fire; it's like trying to describe the scent of human blood dripping into a sandy loamy ground in a distant country. It's like describing the smell of the trapped air in the closed confines of the lost Ark; it's just hard to do.

However, the smell of disease is quite different.

The abdominal cavity does a great job of containing and hiding the stench of disease until the cavity is opened. The longer the time between the start of the disease and entering the abdominal cavity, the more intense the smell. Opening the diseased but undiagnosed abdominal cavity, is like taking the lid off a garbage can containing table scraps, egg shells, spilt milk, a dead rat, and some old fish; the longer the lid is closed, the more intense, disgusting, and offensive the odor of the trapped fetid air.

According to Georgia's history, her perforation occurred right after her lunch at 12:30. I first examined her around 8pm, so now, at 9pm, over eight hours had passed since the disease began. It takes less than an hour for leaking intestinal contents to develop enough bacterial gases to fill the abdominal cavity with putrid odors; odors strong enough overcome the most experienced and hardened OR member's olfactory capacity resulting in multiple members gagging and vomiting. This is why each member, before entering the OR room, applied a small amount of liquid peppermint, menthol, eucalyptus oil, and lemon to their masks. This combination oil compound, like a witch's incanted brew, wards off offensive smells and, in the battle of odors, defeats the evil vapors by a defense wall of sweet, powerful, perfumed effluvium.

By definition, a perforated abdominal organ means a hollow organ. A spleen or a liver can rupture but not perforate; they are solid organs, not hollow. The hollow organs or viscus in the abdomen are esophagus, stomach, small and large intestines, gallbladder, urinary bladder, uterus, and fallopian tubes. One of these eight organs had a hole in it.

Dr. Isaiah Sampson delivered Patsy and two days later, delivered Georgia's uterus as well. It was a full term, uncomplicated pregnancy and Georgia and Gabriel planned many more. Before the pregnancy, in the early mornings, before the jealous sunlight, before the night's candles burned out and the happy day peeped over the foggy mountain tops, they lay close against each other and whispered in the darkness. This was their time. It was the time when nothing else mattered, nothing else intervened, nothing else pulled them apart; it was the time of Patsy's conception. Georgia and Gabriel talked of dreams and desires and destiny. In soft murmurings, in soothing words, sounds barely heard through lips brushing against naked skin, they confessed to each other visions of future moments, future celebrations, and future birthdays of all their many running, laughing, jumping, giggling, climbing, singing children. Dr. Sampson knew nothing of this. He only saw a young nineteen year old girl continuously bleeding from a torn, ripped, and mangled postpartum uterus. His choice was easy; hers was not.

Georgia and Gabriel had no time for their predawn Shakespearean intimacy. Dr. Sampson did not give them the opportunity to discuss their decision in their secretive, protected, and undisturbed chamber; she was bleeding, he could not stop it, he had no compatible blood to transfuse, he had no time to waste. When gray haired, white-coated, bow-tied Dr. Sampson entered the hospital room, he didn't have to ask the question; Gabriel gave the answer.

"We have decided to have the operation. We are ready." Gabriel said without looking at Dr. Sampson. He held Georgia's hand in his right and rubbed her back with his left. She never stopped crying.

At 1:30pm, Eastern Standard Time, on November 22, 1963, while president Kennedy lay dead in a Dallas hospital emergency department, Dr. James Theodor Reckner, family physician in Hyden, Kentucky, placed his last stitch in the skin of Georgia's right upper quadrant after removing her gangrenous infected gallbladder. Georgia always claimed that a part of her died the day Kennedy was shot.

The list of potential perforated organs decreased by three;

the fallopian tubes, although still in her abdomen, cannot perforate unless attached to a uterus; five organs remained.

Two of the five, the small and large intestine, have a combined length of 40 feet. A perforation can occur anywhere along those long entrails; a perforation sometimes no larger than a pencil eraser but just as deadly as the crater left by a 30-30 caliber rifle bullet.

When Angel and I had cut through the thin peritoneum and exposed the abdominal cavity to the outside air and hot lights, we did not expect to find what we immediately found, the released bottle of normal abdominal cavity smell. No pent up, concentrated, augmented malodorous stench of disease erupted up through the small peritoneal hole. Only the distant, distinct, and disturbing smell I knew so well.

Angel looked at me. She leaned over Georgia's open abdomen and whispered to me, "what are we going to do?"

I raised my eyebrows and simply answered, "we search."

"For what?"

"For the hole. It has to be here. The CT scan showed it, my physical exam confirmed it, her lab results supported it, and her vital signs reflected it; it is here." I emphasized the last three words with strong, short, staccato tones. "It could be walled off by some edematous intestine or omentum or mesentery. Maybe it's in the greater omental sac. Maybe it's behind the bladder. Maybe it's a retrocecal appendix. Whatever. But we'll find it and fix it."

After twenty years as a surgeon, most operations are routine and straightforward but a few are not and those few stress and disquiet me and when I am stressed, I loudly, repeatedly, and forcibly blow out inhaled air. I deeply inhale through my mouth with a sucking sound, hold my breath for a few seconds, and then blow out again with a loud swooshing sound; I repeat this process until the stress disappears; the volume and number of cycles is directly proportional to the stress intensity. If I discover the swollen, infected, nearly perforated appendix tightly tucked and hidden underneath the colon instead of dangling totally exposed below the colon, making my laparoscopic removal difficult, tedious, and time consuming, I will softly blow maybe four or five times while working to remove it. If I find a gangrenous, perforated, edematous, rotting gallbladder, an advanced infected state, a condition totally obliterating the normal anatomical borders between the small simple gallbladder duct and the large, dangerous, life essential common bile duct, I will loudly blow countless times until I have safely removed the entire organ.

There is something else that happens during the stressful times, the ghosts appear.

The ghosts always appear when I start to blow. They usually stand just behind Angel's left side. I see them as plain, as clear, as distinct, as they appeared in real life so many years ago. They're dressed in scrubs but not in gowns, or gloves, or masks. They lean over the open abdomen and peer inside or if it's a laparoscopic case, they will look at the video screen. It's always only one ghost, never two or more, but different ghosts appear depending on the stress intensity. After a few seconds, the ghost will look at me and slightly smile(a reassuring, confident, soothing smile). After opening Georgia's abdomen, I looked at Angel and he was standing on her left staring into the open cavity.

"Now Daner. Whenever you're exploring an abdomen for some disease or injury, start looking in the quadrants first." He spoke to me in the soft voice of Dr. Wayne Warrior, one of my past surgical professors, a Vietnam war surgeon, an intense, no nonsense, superbly trained University of Alabama surgeon.

"After you look in and pack off the quadrants, run the bowel Daner. Run the bowel. Start at the ligament of Treitz (muscularius suspensorious duodenum), where the jejunum starts, and work, inch by inch, distally to the ileocecal valve (where the small and large intestine join). Then run the bowel in reverse and repeat. If you don't find the injury in the small intestine, look at the left colon, in the pelvis, and run backwards to the ileocecal valve, reverse, and repeat."

"If you don't find an injury in the large bowel, look for the rare causes. Check out the greater sac, underneath the stomach.

Open the sac and look carefully at the posterior stomach. If that is normal, run the bowel again, both small and large."

"Remember Daner, the obvious injury is not what kills patients; it is the small, subtle, easily overlooked injury that is deadly. Before you give up, double-check everything from urinary bladder to esophagus to rectum. God may be forgiving, but disease and injury is not."

"Okay."

"Okay what?" Angel asked.

"Okay. Lets start in the quadrants."

"Large Ricardson." BJ handed me an instrument similar to a small hand held metal hoe; the six inch long handle attached at a right angle to a thin, flat, wide, blade, was designed to fit snugly under the edge of the abdominal incision or under the ribs allowing the assistant to pull up exposing the anatomical area underneath. Like all retractors, the Richardson has several different sizes from large to small. I placed it under the left upper ribs and Angel pulled up toward the ceiling. With the left upper abdominal wall retracted, I could see the deep red, wedge shaped, blood engorged spleen. I laid my right palm against the back it.

"Remember Daner, the spleen is unlike any other organ; it is fragile, frangible, fracturable." Dr. Warrior's ghost spoke again. "If you pull it, its thin peritoneal capsule will tear, its short stomach veins will rip, its hilum will split and blood will burst out in an unrepairable gush. Push it down only."

I pushed the soft, squishy, lymphatic organ straight down toward Georgia's feet and inspected the area behind it and underneath diaphragm; it was dry, clean, odorless. While holding the spleen down, Georgia's heart beat against the back of my hand, rhythmically bouncing on the trampoline like-diaphragm and slapping my hand like a perpetual living metronome.

"Lap sponge." Jason unraveled and unfurled the flag-like white garment and laid it on the open incision. I grasped it with my left hand, stuffed it into the uncovered space, slowly relaxed my pressure against the spleen and slid my hand free. I took the retractor from Angel.

I stood on Georgia's right side so by holding the retractor in my left hand, I could lift the right side. The giant liver, five times the size of the tenuous spleen, occupied the entire right upper quadrant and spilled over into half of the left upper quadrant. The liver, the largest organ in the cavity, the biggest gland in the body, with a monarch's robe color, an aristocratic, renaissance, enlightenment wonder of functions and roles, awed me as usual with its grand look, indestructible nature, and glistening velvety surface. I tenderly, reverently, slid my right hand over its smooth, sensual, satiny figure, enjoying the tactile titillation of touching a sovereign body.

Above it, I saw nothing but the respiratory flattening and retracting of the right sided diaphragm. Under it, in a cradled bed where the robins egg blue gallbladder once slept, a portion of adherent omentum, the fat filled curtain draping over all of the cavity contents, obliterated this space below the liver's under edge, on top of the right kidney, and above the crossing tunnel of large intestine; a consequence of Dr. Reckner's operation. This space, filled now with scar, is Morison's (British surgeon) pouch. It too was devoid of any abnormal smell, fluid, disease; I stuffed another lap sponge here.

"Okay Sonya, Trendelenburg (German surgeon)." Sonya pushed the table's electric positioning device and the table smoothly positioned Georgia's body with her head down toward the floor and her feet up in the air. This arrangement utilized gravity to shift the internal organs, specifically the intestines, out of the pelvis and up against the diaphragm. Now the lower quadrants opened to me.

"Retractor to Angel". BJ handed it to her. "Lets look in the left side first."

She pulled upward; I pushed my left hand against the colon and slowly pressed down revealing the space on top of the lower sigmoid colon where it disappears underneath the reflection of peritoneum. Above this peritoneal reflection, a space once existed between the sigmoid and the underside of the uterus, Douglas (Scottish physician) pouch, but due to the saving surgery of

Dr. Sampson, this space is occupied by filmy, transparent, wisps of scar called adhesions. Again, an area usually filled with the drippings, dregs, and debris of perforation, remained crystal clear. I packed another lap sponge, took the retractor again, and said, “Lets look on the right.”

The usual suspect for criminal activity in the right pelvis is the vermiform appendix; the Satan of the body cavity. The serpent in the garden of anatomical perfection; a more maligned, malicious, and malevolent organ has never existed. Deceptively adept at delaying detection and diagnosis of disease, the appendix is infamous. Unlike other common diseases, like strep throat, flu, hepatitis, pneumonia, kidney infection, heart attack, there is no diagnostic test available to definitively discover appendicitis; finding it is always a combination of high suspicion and guess work.

Appendicitis is the master mimicker; every symptom it causes is common and usual for a host of other diseases. Right lower quadrant pain is produced by kidney stones, ovarian cysts, trapped gas, colon spasm, viral infections, Crohn’s (American physician) disease, constipation and more. All of these maladies, except kidney stones, can cause tenderness, fever, and elevated white cell count. All of them cause nausea, vomiting, diarrhea, and appetite suppression, just like acute appendicitis; nothing is unique for appendicitis.

The appendix is a small, wormy, short, pencil shaped vestigial nothing of an organ, an insignificant afterthought of evolution, a useless intestinal tonsil of tissue, a remnant of some prehistoric benefit, and a murderer of human beings. An appendiceal perforation, an inevitable consequence of undiagnosed acute appendicitis, transforms an insignificant remnant of an organ, into a hellish, vicious, diabolical organic perpetrator of infectious mayhem, chaos, disaster, and horrific death. The feces, intestinal fluid, bacteria, blood, and pus leaking from a disintegrated appendix into the sterile sanctity of the peritoneal cavity is like a burst sewage line spewing spoilage into the oak barrel of fermenting French Merlot.

Georgia's appendix dangled into the pelvis two inches. Its pale white, smooth, shiny, thin serosal surface healthily reflected the OR lights; no disease had ever occupied its small normal lumen. Like on the left side, the right ovary was a shriveled, ghastly remnant of lost, pathetically unused fertility. Each fallopian tube drooped lazily down into the flimsy scar left by Dr. Sampson; each a cobwebbed, deserted, desecrated, destitute, disconnected tunnel of fecundity.

"Lets run the bowel. Angel, start at the ligament."

Running the bowel is a surgical term of unknown etymology but it doesn't accurately describe the procedure. Starting at the ligament of Treitz, where the duodenum (first part of the small intestine just past the stomach) ends and the rest of the small intestine begins, the first assistant squeezes the bowel with her fingers while I squeeze the bowel a few inches from her. The five inch long segment of intestine between us is what we 'run' or look at, inspect, and manipulate. We scrutinize the complete circumference of the bowel, even the lower edge where the blood vessels pierce the bowel. If a hole exists, no matter how small, it will leak out bilious, yellow-green, intestinal fluid. Squeezing increases the luminal pressure, squirting fluid out, staining the exposed bowel, and marking the perforation.

We move down the small intestine in five-inch increments until we reach the ileocecal valve; we did not find any intestinal fluid, any blood, or any holes. We reverse the process and work the five-inch segments back to the ligament; still no holes.

"Lets repeat it." We do the entire double run again with the same result.

"Okay. Lets do the large intestine." Running the large intestine is slower and more difficult even though the large intestine is only five feet long as compared to the 32-foot long small intestine. The large intestine on the right and left side reposes naked in the peritoneal cavity, visible, unprotected and easily examined with little manipulation, but the omentum completely covers the transverse colon, the part crossing from one side to the other. The omentum, packed with fat, lymphatic tissue, and blood vessels, seeks, senses, and secures itself to diseased or injured organs and temporarily stanches the leaking fluid.

I slid both my hands along the large intestine starting on the right side where the appendix comes out and the small intestine comes in, and followed it up to below the liver, where the colon turns left and becomes the omentum covered transverse colon. I grab the thick twelve inch wide tissue and flip it up to assess the transverse colon's sides and bottom. In the left upper quadrant, where the spleen resides, the omentum ends and the now naked colon curves down as the descending colon. Half-way down the left colon, it curves gently to the right and then back to the left forming an S-shaped part called the sigmoid. All along this segment, partially obscured by the blood vessels feeding the colon, small, fingertip sized bulges and bumps project up off the wall like spaced Braille letters. These Braille like structures, scattered and sown on the colon wall like hand tossed grain seeds, are hollow pouches connected to the colon lumen by tiny openings.

These openings appear as mucosal holes when visualized by the colonoscope and change the normal, smooth, unblemished colon mucosa into moon-like craters. Each crater marks a passageway into the Braille- like hollow pouches called diverticula. These diverticula are notorious causes of infection, inflammation, bleeding, blockages, and perforations. Caused by an American fast food diet low in fiber and nutrition, exacerbated by the American epidemic of constipation, and irritated by any food particle small enough to lodge and block the crater entrance, they start forming in a person's twenties and multiply with age. A dozen of them populated Georgia's 79 year old colon; all were small, short, uninflamed, uninfected, and unconcerning. None of them had ever been infected much less perforated or abscessed.

"What now?" whispered Angel?

"The greater sac and the esophagus." I look at her staring at me with a questioning, worried look about her blue eyes. "We will find it Angel. Sonya, reverse Trendelenburg please." The table smoothly moved into the new position.

"Babcock." BJ passed a hemostat looking instrument with smooth, non-crushing tips designed by the American surgeon, Wayne Babcock. I used them to grasp the lower or greater stomach curvature and then handed it to Angel. While she lifted up on the stomach border, I pulled the lower tissue down. Behind this area of tissue tension was a space underneath the stomach called the greater sac. In this space, a perforated posterior stomach ulcer would be found.

"Cautery." Angel handed me the pencil-like device used to turn electrical energy into heat. I cauterized a hole in the tissue and peeped beneath the stomach; nothing. It was dry, devoid of any pathology. I removed the Babcock clamp, placed my left hand on the front surface of the stomach and pulled it down toward her feet. Now I could see the junction between the stomach and esophagus; nothing again. No esophageal hole.

I looked at Angel but the ghost was gone.

"Lets check each quadrant." I removed each lap sponge from the quadrants but all were clean and dry.

Sonya peeped over the sterile drape and looked at the open cavity. She said nothing. Bj, Shana, and Jason remained silent. "What's next Dana?" Angel asked softly. I looked at her again but the ghost was back.

"Daner, negative laparotomies are as rare as hen's teeth and most are normal because the surgeon overlooked something. Are you sure you haven't missed something?"

"Yes, I'm sure." I whispered.

"What?" asked Angel.

"Nothing. Just talking to myself. "I audibly exhaled and stepped away from the table. I paced a few times.

"Shana. Pull up the CT scan from the emergency department."

She typed on the keyboard and the black and white images popped up.

"Scroll down Shana." I said as I leaned over her shoulder. She moved the images down the numbered sequence. "Stop."

Each number on the image represented a 0.5cm slice of

Georgia's body and starting at image 46 through image 54, a total body length of thirteen cm, the gray images showed a thickening of the sigmoid colon with fluid and air outside the colon.

"Shana read me the radiologist's report."

She found the faxed report in the paper chart. "Inflammatory changes in the descending and sigmoid colon with moderate amount of fluid and free air compatible and worrisome for an inflamed and ruptured viscus, probably a diverticulum, with signs of peritonitis. Clinical correlation recommended."

"Okay. Read the name of the patient, birthdate, and social on the report and on the x-ray images." She read them off; they were identical to Georgia's wrist band.

"Date? Look at the date on the images and on the report." She did. They were correct; no clerical error existed.

"Shana. Call X-ray and ask them to call the radiologist and have her call me in here." Shana dialed the extension.

"Hey Brandon. This is Shana Crawford in OR B. Dr. Edwards needs to talk with the radiologist that is reading tonight. Could you get her and connect her to us? Thanks." She didn't wait for a response , she just hung up. I paced and exhaled. Seconds seemed like hours. Finally the phone rang.

"Hello. This is OR B. Is this Dr. Henson?" Silence. "Okay. Thank you Dr. Henson. I have Dr. Edwards and he needs to talk with you. Hold just a moment. She's on the line Dr. Edwards."

"Put her on speaker."

"Hold on Dr. Henson, I'm putting you on speaker."

"Hey Dr. Henson, this is Dana Edwards."

"Hey Dr. Edwards. This is Kamille Henson. How can I help you?"

"I'm operating on Georgia Conway. You read her CT scan of the abdomen and pelvis with contrast a few hours ago and I just have a question for you please."

"Sure. I have her films up. Go ahead."

"Your report indicated free air, inflammation, and peritonitis. Would you look at the scan again and give me your interpretation again?"

"Sure. I'm reviewing the images now. There is definitely free air, actually a lot of free air, under the left and right diaphragms. Along the left gutter about midway down the descending colon, is a considerable amount of edema and reactive inflammatory changes in the mesocolon and down in the pelvis there is a considerable amount of fluid compatible with leakage of intestinal contents and subsequent peritonitis. Does that help you?"

"Yes Dr. Henson. That helps. Thank you for calling in. I hope the rest of your evening is quiet."

"Okay. No problem. I hope your patient does well. Good night." Shana disconnected the speaker. The room was quiet. Nobody looked at me or at each other.

I looked at Angel. No ghost. A surgeon once told me all surgeons are products of their training. Not a very profound saying but certainly a vague saying. What I think is more accurate is that surgeons, all surgeons, are imitators of the men and women who trained them. Not imitators of just one surgeon, or one specific professor; but an amalgamation of all of them. A composite. I'm not just like Dr. Wayne Warrior but rather I'm somewhat like him and somewhat like Dr. Tom Rock and Dr. David Tiller and Dr. Joe Good and Dr. Lisa McCoy and Dr. Beth Lambert and Dr. Paul Blanton and Dr. William Bowman. And each of them are composites of their professors. Like a genetic heritage in a family, each surgeon carries the genes of skill, technique, diagnostic acumen, and professional attitude. All of these surgeon genes come from the ancestors of the profession; the men and women innovators, researchers, and avant-garde surgeons who were the firsts. These include Dr. Claudius Amyand, the French surgeon who in 1735 successfully removed the first appendix; Dr. Christian Barnard, the South African who performed the first heart transplantation in 1967; Dr. William DeVries, the American who implanted the first artificial heart in 1982; Dr. John Gibbon, the American who performed the first open heart surgery in 1953. The list would include Joseph Lister, John Hunter, Harvey Cushing, Michael DeBakey, Denton Cooley, Thomas Starzl, William Halstead, and dozens more; and all of them share a common attribute; they were all pioneers, all trailblazers, all discovers, and all important to me. All are ghosts in my operating room.

I looked at Angel again. He was there, like always, just behind her left shoulder.

“Dana? What are you going to do?” Angel asked me. I blew out and walked back to the table.

“Daner. Always remember the most important truth about surgery. Never forget, not ever, that surgeons treat patients, not X-rays, not labs, not CT scans. Daner, look at your patient and learn the truth.”

“BJ?”

“Yes sir.”

“Jason.”

“Yes sir.”

“Sponge count.”

“Yes sir.” They responded in unison.

“Angel.”

“Dana.”

“Lets close.”

“Shana.”

“Yessir.”

“What’s in that CD player on your desk?”

“Excuse me Dr. Edwards? Did you say CD player?”

Everyone stopped and looked at me. “Yes. I said CD player. Play anything you want.”

“Uh, yes sir.”

“And Shana. Play it loud.”

“Yessir. Do you have a preference?”

I thought for just a moment. “Only one. For God’s sake, don’t play Don Giovanni.”

CONTENTS

EPILOGUE

I performed another colonoscopy on Carolyn Kingston six months later; it was as normal as the last one. Every year for the past five years, I have repeated her colonoscopy; all have been normal. A year ago, she self-published her account of what happened.

Georgia Conway went home six days after her surgery. She never experienced another episode of severe abdominal pain, never came back to the emergency department and as far as I know, she never talked with Dr. Quinton again. She lived for many years and spent every moment with Patsy.

Made in United States
North Haven, CT
11 May 2025

68752089R10053